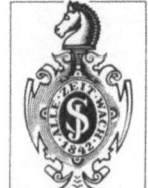

M. Paneth · P. Goldstraw · B. Hyams

Fundamental Techniques in Pulmonary and Oesophageal Surgery

With 262 Illustrations

Springer-Verlag
London Berlin Heidelberg New York
Paris Tokyo

Matthias Paneth, FRCS
Consultant Cardiothoracic Surgeon, The Brompton Hospital, Fulham Road, London SW3 6HP

Peter Goldstraw, FRCS
Consultant Cardiothoracic Surgeon, The Brompton Hospital, Fulham Road, London SW3 6HP

Barbara Hyams, MA, AMI,
Medical Illustrator, Poynings, Northchurch Common, Northchurch, Berkhamsted,
Hertfordshire

ISBN-13: 978-1-4471-3124-3   e-ISBN-13: 978-1-4471-3122-9
DOI: 10.1007/978-1-4471-3122-9

British Library Cataloguing in Publication Data
Paneth, M.
Fundamental techniques in pulmonary and oesophageal surgery.
1. Lungs – Surgery   2. Esophagus – Surgery   I. Title   II. Goldstraw, P.   III. Hyams, Barbara E.
617′.542   RD 539

Library of Congress Cataloging-in-Publication Data
Paneth, M. (Matthias), 1921–
Fundamental techniques in pulmonary and oesophageal surgery.
Includes bibliographies and index.
1. Lungs – Surgery. 2. Esophagus – Surgery. I. Goldstraw, P. (Peter), 1945–   . II. Hyams, B. (Barbara),
1950–   . III. Title. [DNLM: 1. Esophagus – surgery. 2. Lung – surgery. WF 668 P191f] RD539.P36
1987 617′.542 87–9523

© Springer-Verlag Berlin Heidelberg 1987
Softcover reprint of the hardcover 1st edition 1987

Filmset and printed by BAS Printers Limited, Over Wallop, Hampshire

2128/3916 543210

Preface

This book sets out to illustrate the key steps in some of the commoner procedures in pulmonary and oesophageal surgery. Each chapter deals with one operation. It was always our intention that the emphasis should be on detailed illustrations of the various stages of each operation. The text is of secondary importance, serving to provide continuity and to guide the reader through the illustrations.

The techniques outlined are those which have evolved in our practice over the years and are therefore the result of varied influences and personal experience. Where an individual surgeon's name is attached to an operative technique we make no claim to describe the procedure exactly as that surgeon would have performed it, and it would perhaps have been more accurate to describe the technique as being "in the style of . . . . . .". We would wish to apologise in advance to any surgeon who feels that we have not accurately depicted his technique or have deviated from it in any important respect.

The book is intended to complement and in no way to form an alternative to formal surgical apprenticeship: there can be no substitute for assisting an experienced surgeon and having him assist the trainee. We hope, however, that it will be of assistance to the young surgeon setting out on a career in this speciality. It will allow him at his leisure to preview the steps to be undertaken in the proposed operation and complement his observations in the operating theatre. The experienced surgeon may find it of assistance as a quick résumé when faced with an operation that he has not performed for some time. We believe that such a reader may find the details of the surgical steps helpful, even if he does not follow each illustration faithfully in his own practice.

It has not been our intention to cover in detail the indications for the operations, nor to outline the pre-operative selection of patients with pulmonary or oesophageal disease. We have made no mention of post-operative complications, and only the briefest of comments on post-operative management.

We may be criticised for our choice of operations to be illustrated. The choice has been a personal one, and we have deliberately omitted operations such as thoracoplasty and segmental resection, which are being performed with decreasing frequency, and operations such as those on the trachea and chest wall, where we feel that patients should be treated in specialist units.

We would like to express our gratitude to and admiration of Barbara Hyams, the illustrator and our collaborator in this project; such value as the book may achieve will mainly be due to the technique and expertise of her detailed illustrations. Many surgeons have influenced the development of these operations and have had a profound impact on our personal techniques. It would be invidious to name any particular surgeons, but we would like to pay tribute to Lord Brock and Mr. Andrew Logan, who have influenced generations of surgeons on either side of the Anglo-Scottish border. We would like to thank our secretaries, Mrs. J. Matthew and Mrs. J. Field, for patiently translating our thoughts and amendments into structured text. As always, the brunt of our literary frustrations has fallen upon our wives and families, and we wish to thank them for their patience, support and understanding.

London, 1987

M. Paneth
P. Goldstraw

Contents

1 Mediastinoscopy 2

2 Mediastinotomy 6

3 Left Thoracotomy 8

4 Right Thoracotomy 18

5 Right Upper Lobectomy 28

6 Right Lower Lobectomy 36

7 Right Middle Lobectomy 42

8 Right Middle and Lower Lobectomy 48

9 Left Lower Lobectomy 54

10 Left Upper Lobectomy 62

11 Right Radical Pneumonectomy 68

12 Left Radical Pneumonectomy 76

13 Sleeve Resection 84

14 Empyema—Decortication 92

15 Hiatus Hernia 96

16 Colon Interposition 110

17 Achalasia 122

18 Leiomyoma 126

19 Carcinoma: Left-Sided Approach for Resection of the Lower Oesophagus
    and Gastro-oesophageal Junction (Logan Operation) 130

20 Carcinoma: Oesophageal Resection from the Right (McKeown Operation) 142

21 Carcinoma: Substernal Gastric Bypass 152

Fundamental Techniques in
Pulmonary and Oesophageal Surgery

1 Mediastinoscopy

Mediastinoscopy is an endoscopic examination of the superior mediastinum through a cervical incision. It allows examination and biopsy of the lymphatic chains around the trachea, both paratracheal chains and those at the main carina. As these gland groups are commonly involved by carcinoma of the bronchus ascending through the mediastinum, mediastinoscopy may be used to obtain tissue diagnosis in advanced carcinomas of the lung or to assess the extent of nodal involvement, which many surgeons feel is important in deciding on the desirability of resection. Mediastinoscopy also permits examination of other structures within the superior mediastinum which may be directly invaded by tumours of the upper lobe, and hence may help in deciding upon the resectability of the condition.

This technique demands total familiarity with the anatomy of the superior mediastinum. The biopsies are taken from lymph nodes intimately associated with such important structures as the aortic arch and head vessels, the superior vena cava and the left recurrent laryngeal nerve. The pleura may be breached, particularly on the right, posterior to the superior vena cava. With experience, however, complications are few and limited to the occurrence of small haematomata and occasional superficial wound infections. In the hands of an experienced surgeon this investigative procedure may be safely undertaken in the presence of superior vena caval obstruction.

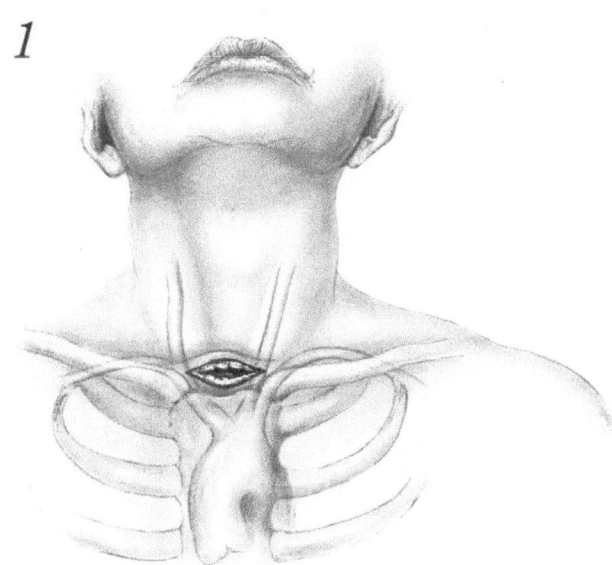

1 The incision is made just above the top of the manubrium, transverse in the midline. The anterior jugular veins may need tying and dividing.

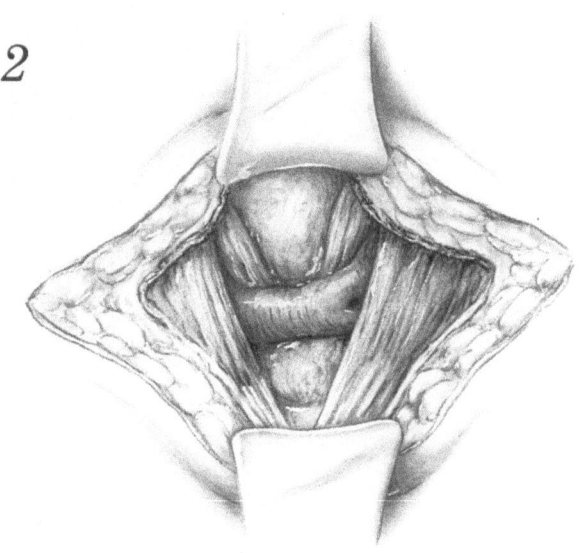

2 The incision is deepened, the venous arch between the anterior jugular veins may be tied and divided and, after the strap muscles have been separated, the trachea is exposed below the thyroid isthmus.

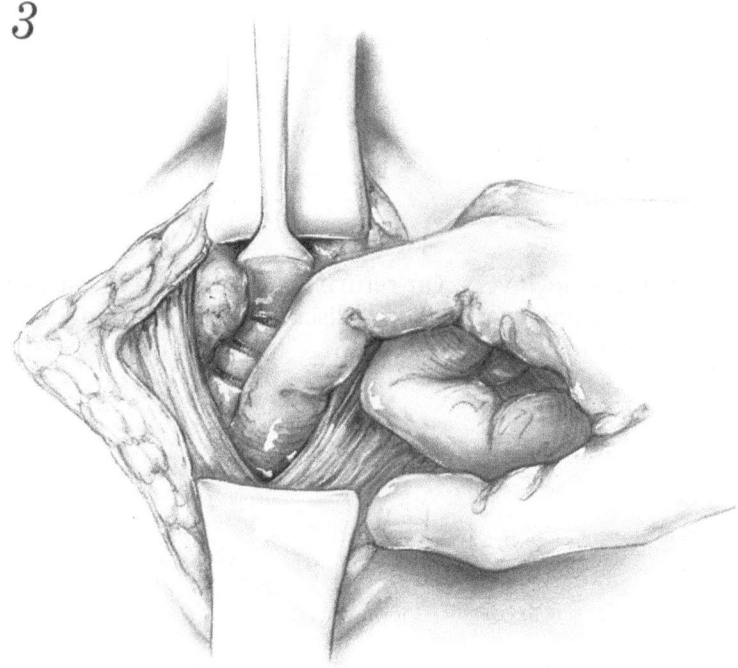

3 The index finger is inserted between the trachea and pretracheal fascia, creating a tunnel behind the brachiocephalic vessels.

4

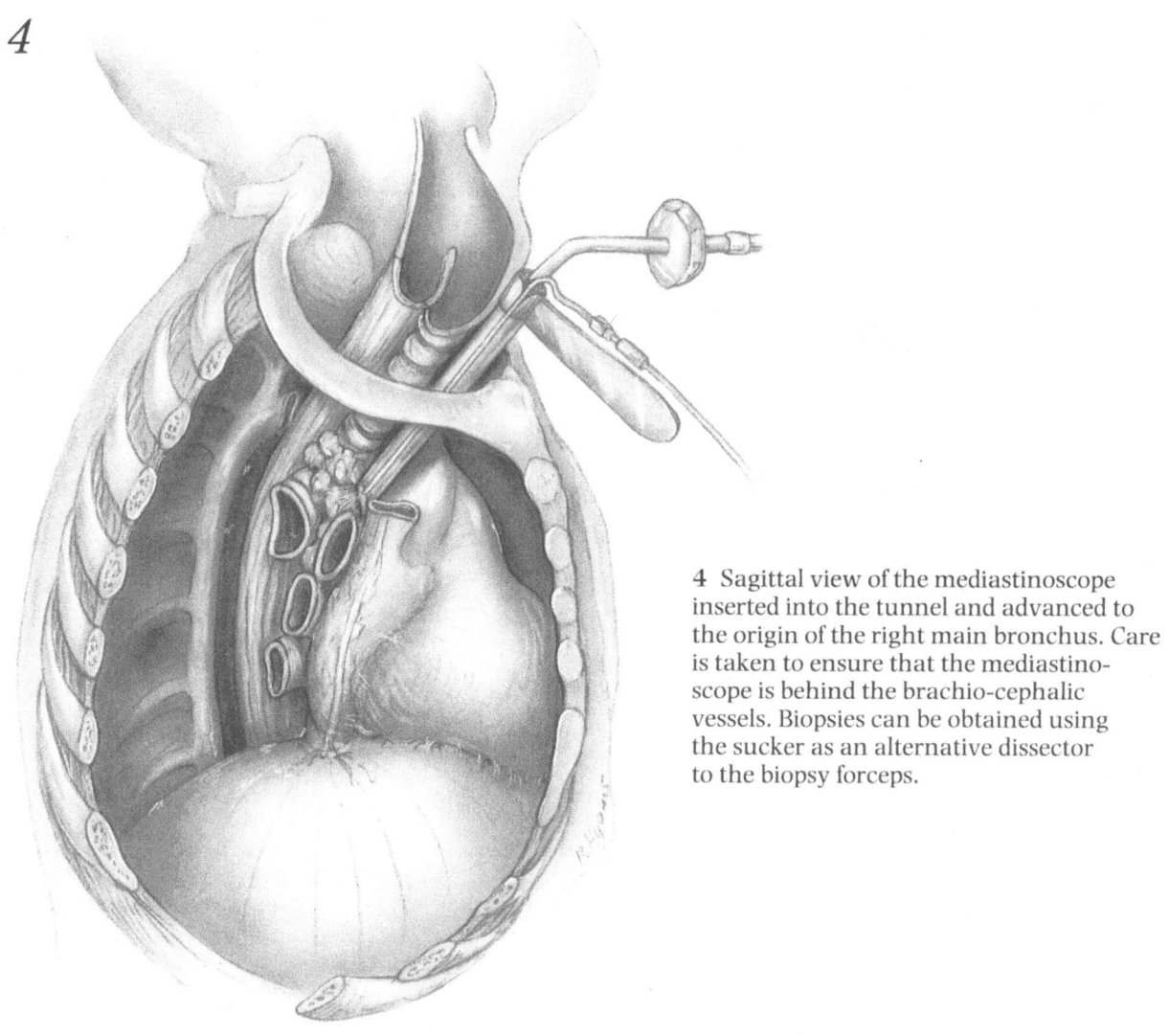

4 Sagittal view of the mediastinoscope inserted into the tunnel and advanced to the origin of the right main bronchus. Care is taken to ensure that the mediastinoscope is behind the brachio-cephalic vessels. Biopsies can be obtained using the sucker as an alternative dissector to the biopsy forceps.

The incision is usually closed without drainage in layers. On return to the ward a chest x-ray should be taken to exclude a pneumothorax. There may be some discomfort on swallowing for 24 h, during which time the patient may prefer to remain on liquids.

2 Mediastinotomy

The short anterior incision provides access to the anterior mediastinum to either side of the sternum. Structures at risk—the internal mammary vessels and the pleura—are troublesome but not crucial. The incision provides a good access to biopsy anterior mediastinal masses. A deeper exploration on the left allows an examination of the subaortic fossa and lymph nodes around the aortic arch—features which may be important when deciding upon the resectability of carcinomas originating in the left upper lobe. The subaortic fossa is palpated digitally. Biopsies should only be taken in this region if histology is essential, since the left recurrent laryngeal nerve is at risk, as are the aorta and pulmonary vessels.

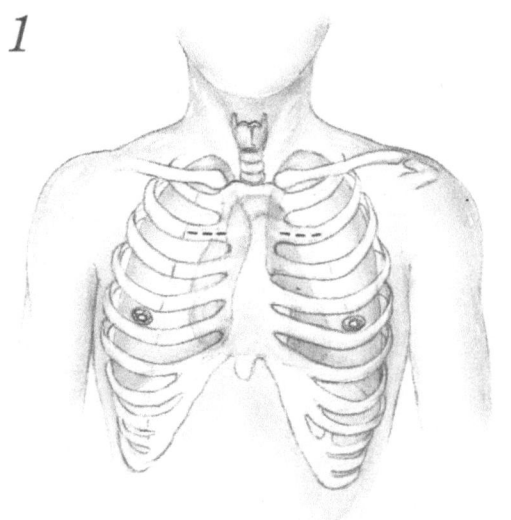

1

1 The incision is centred on the second or third costal cartilages.

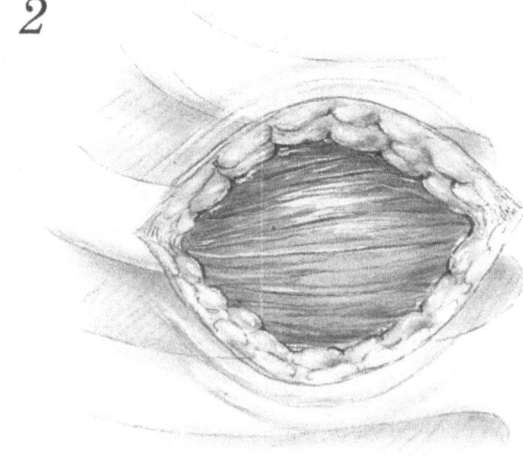

2

2 The incision is deepened to the fibres of the pectoral muscles.

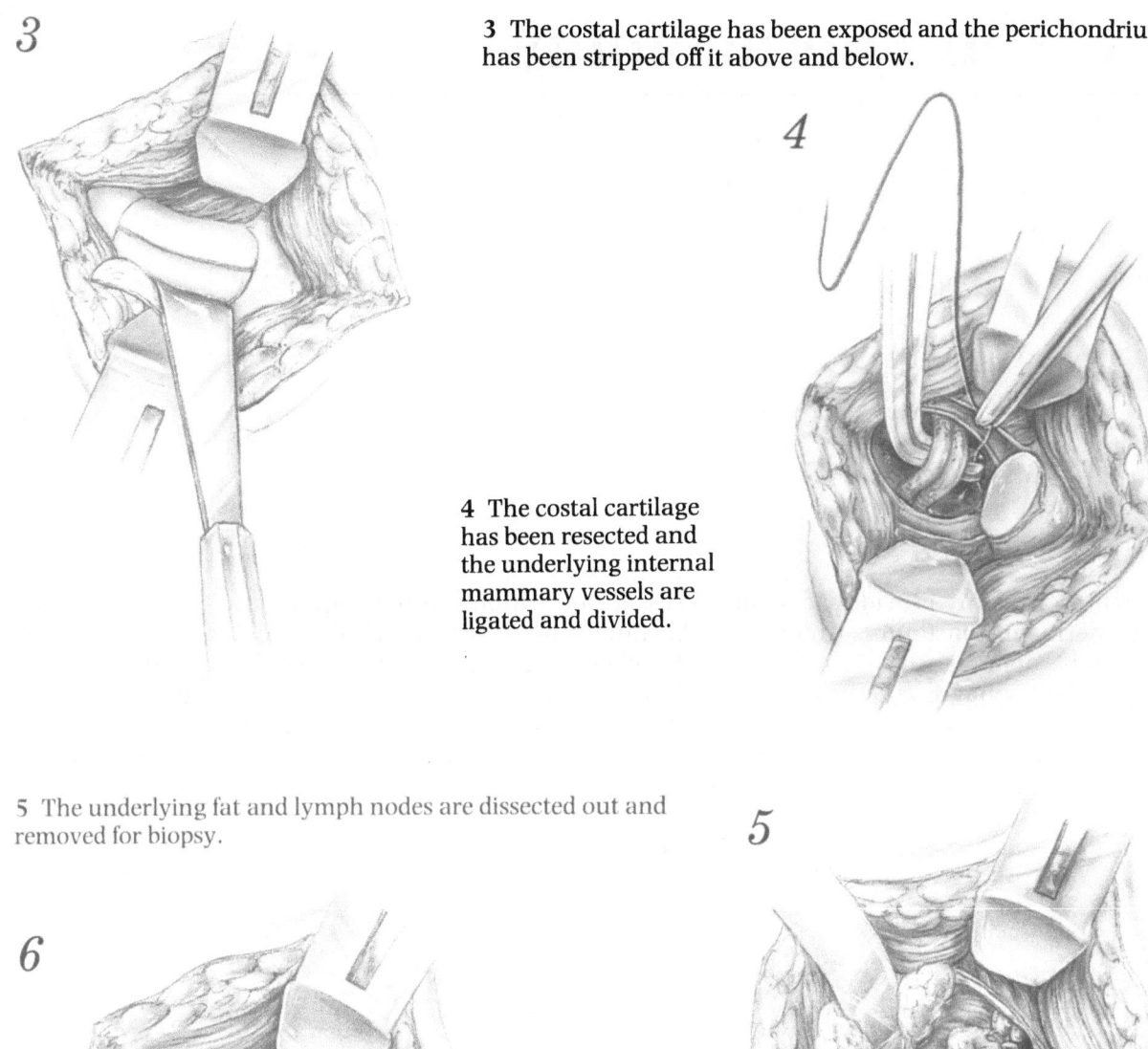

3

3 The costal cartilage has been exposed and the perichondrium has been stripped off it above and below.

4

4 The costal cartilage has been resected and the underlying internal mammary vessels are ligated and divided.

5 The underlying fat and lymph nodes are dissected out and removed for biopsy.

5

6

6 A similar view for the left side.

The incision is closed in layers, usually without drainage. If the pleura has been opened a small drain may be left in place during closure to remove trapped air and removed at the end of the operation.

On return to the ward a chest x-ray should be taken to exclude a pneumothorax.

3 Left Thoracotomy

Left thoractomy provides adequate access for operations on the left lung and the left side of the posterior mediastinum. Anterior mediastinal masses with marked asymmetry to the left may also be approached by this incision. Excellent access is afforded to the descending aorta, the lower oesophagus and the oesophageal hiatus. Individual surgeons may vary the precise position of the incision but they have in common the division of the extra-thoracic muscle to mobilise the scapula and hence expose the thoracic cage. The muscle division is undertaken low so as to denervate as little of the extra-thoracic muscles as possible.

1

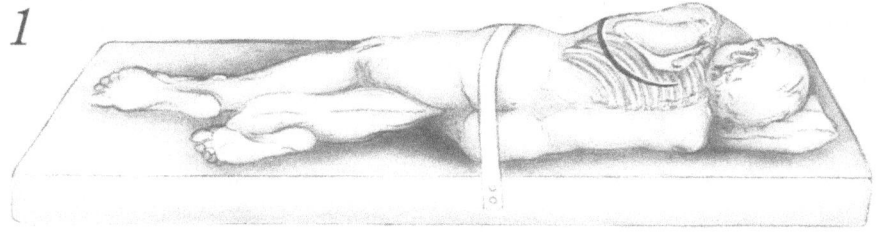

1 The incision in relation to the scapula and ribs is shown from the back. The posterior superior limit of the incision for a standard posterolateral thoracotomy extends to midway between the thoracic spinous processes and the spine of the scapula.

2

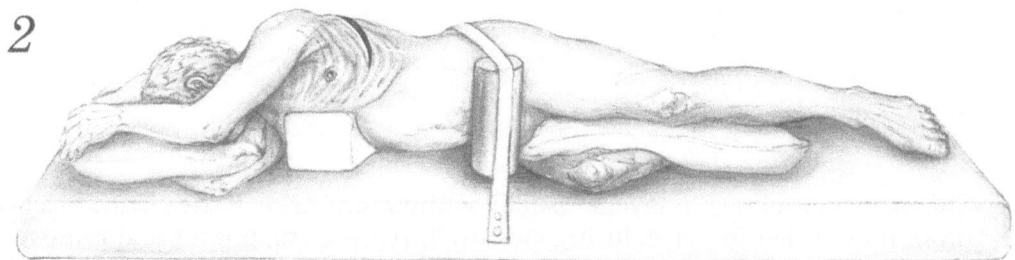

2 The anterior limit of the incision over the sixth or fifth costo-chondral junction.

3

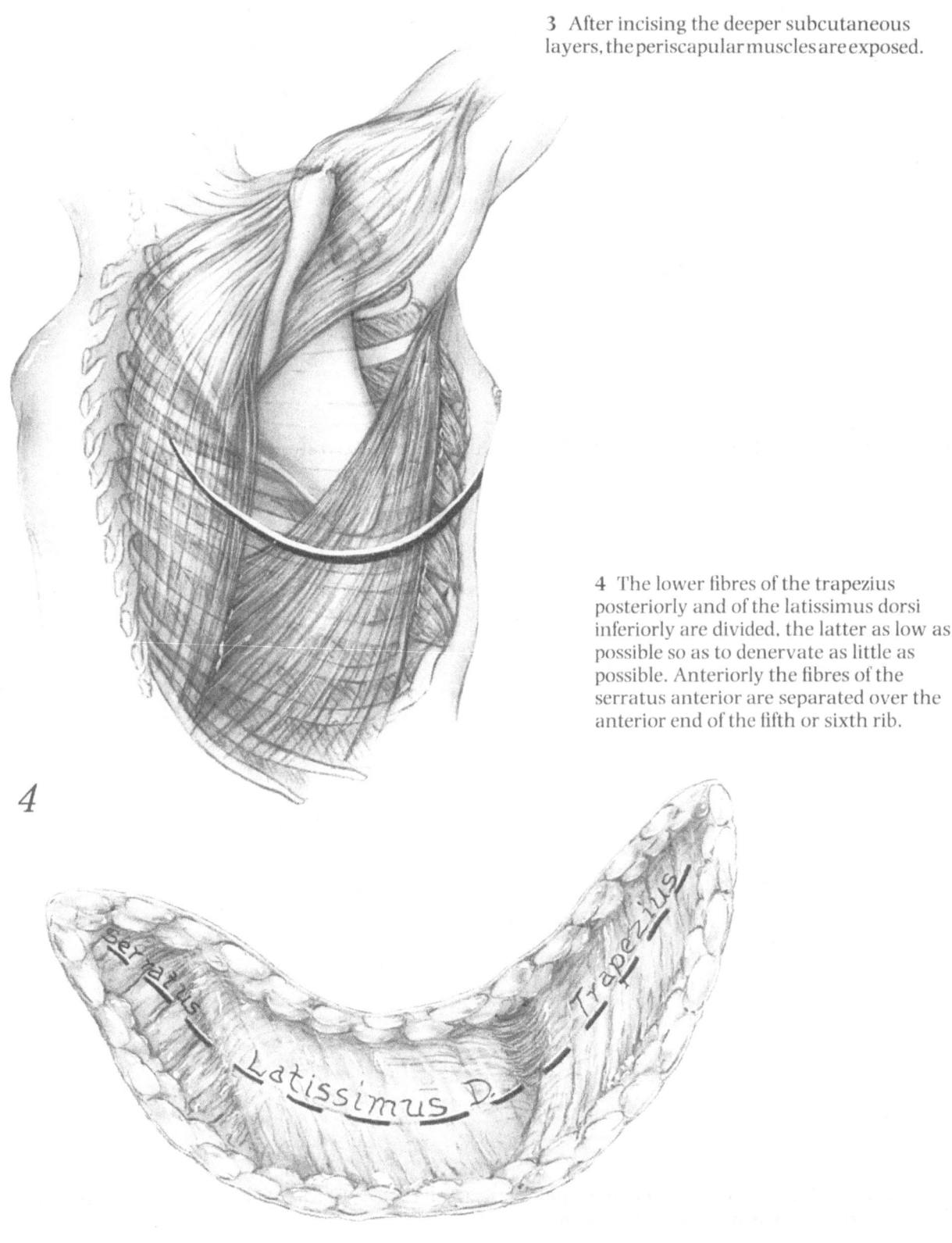

3 After incising the deeper subcutaneous layers, the periscapular muscles are exposed.

4 The lower fibres of the trapezius posteriorly and of the latissimus dorsi inferiorly are divided, the latter as low as possible so as to denervate as little as possible. Anteriorly the fibres of the serratus anterior are separated over the anterior end of the fifth or sixth rib.

4

Serratus — Latissimus D. — Trapezius

5

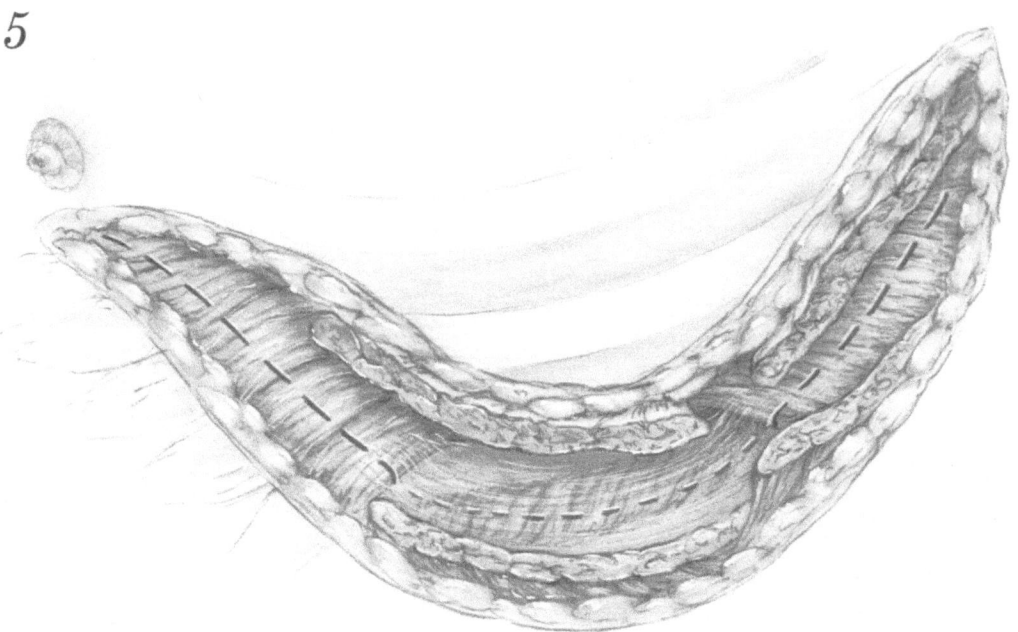

5 Posteriorly the rhomboids are divided in the same plane as the serratus anterior in front.

6

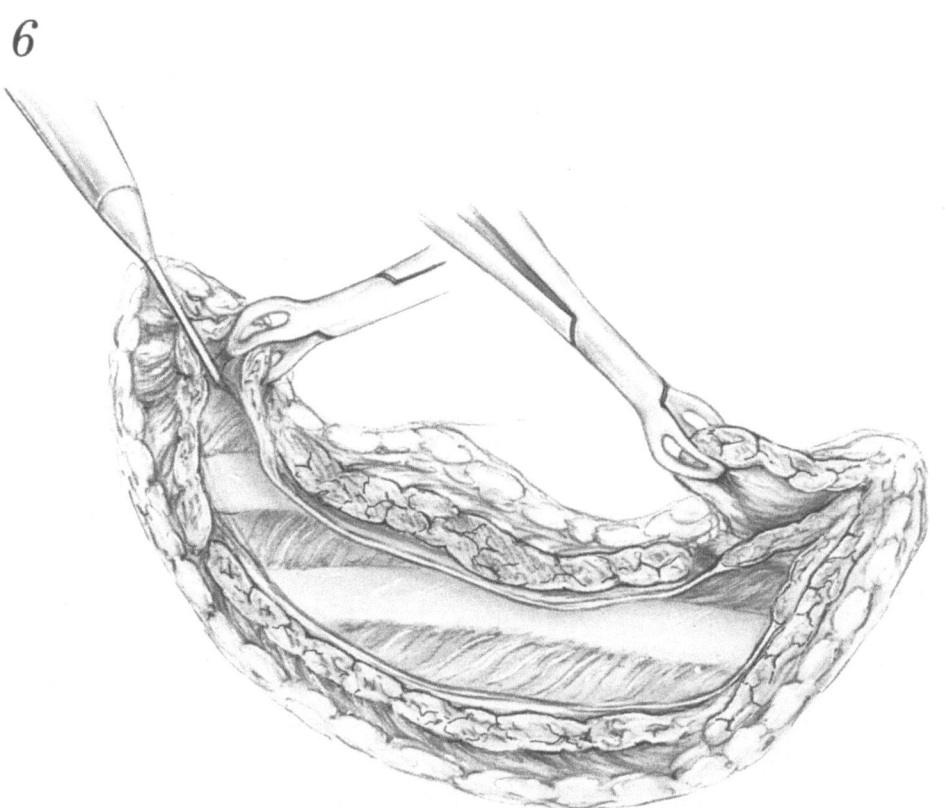

6 Between these two muscles the subscapular fascia is dissected off so as to interfere as little as possible with post-operative movement of the scapula.

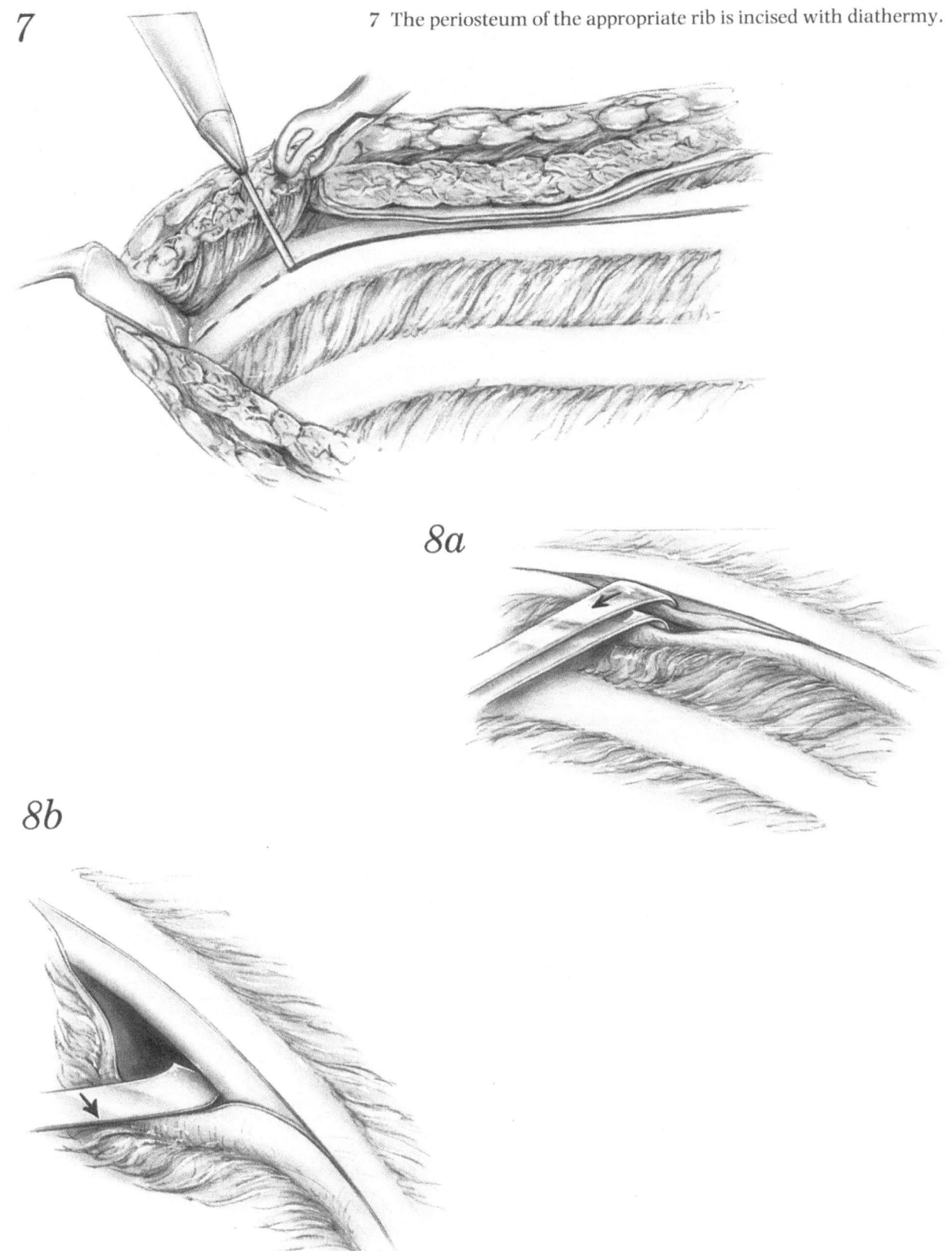

7

7 The periosteum of the appropriate rib is incised with diathermy.

8a

8b

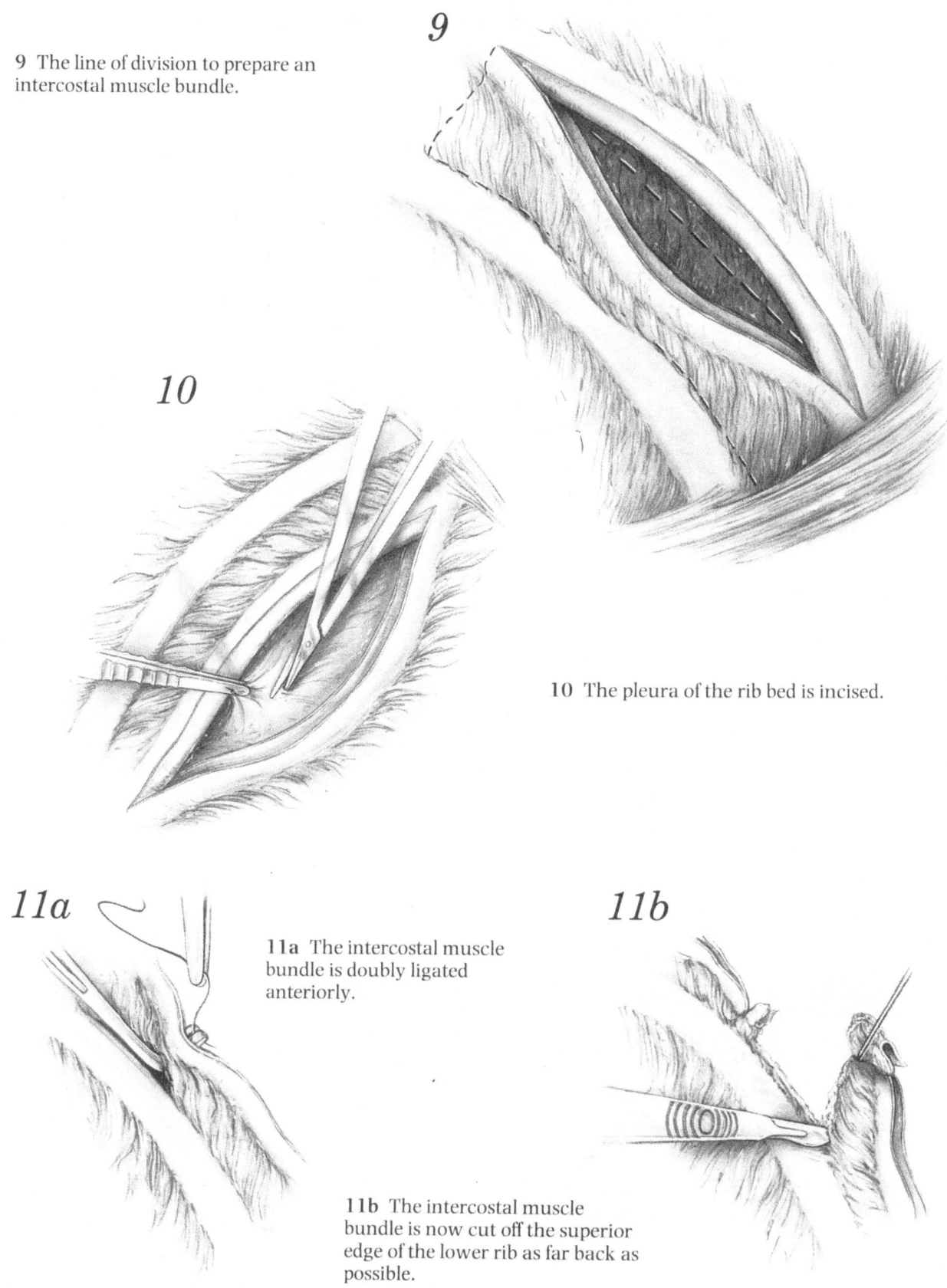

9 The line of division to prepare an intercostal muscle bundle.

10 The pleura of the rib bed is incised.

11a The intercostal muscle bundle is doubly ligated anteriorly.

11b The intercostal muscle bundle is now cut off the superior edge of the lower rib as far back as possible.

12a

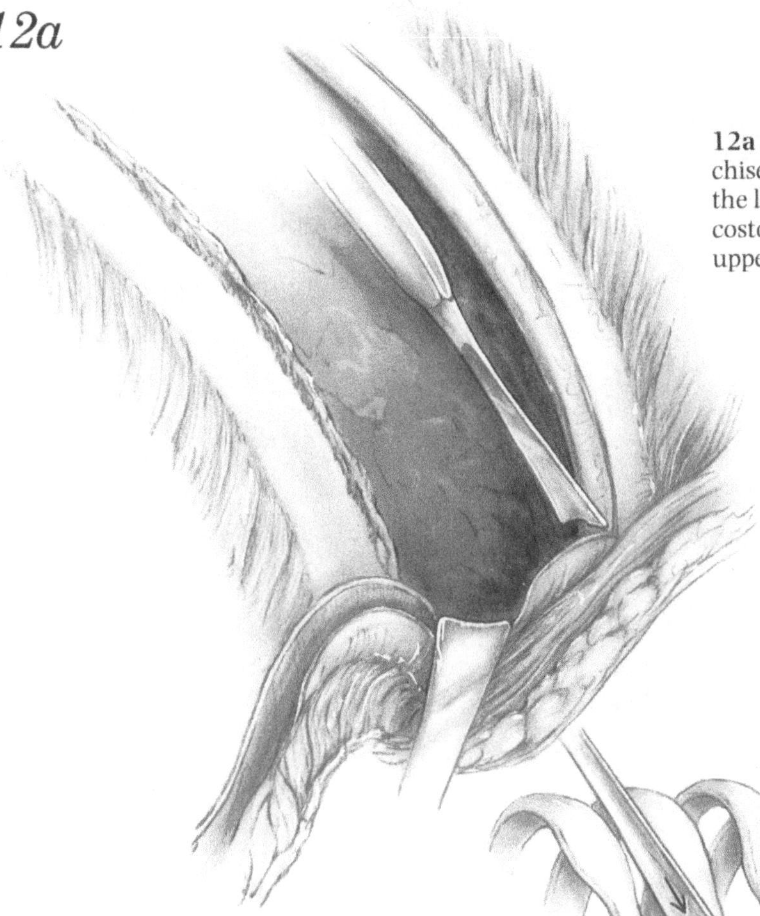

12a The bundle is protected and the Semb chisel is inserted under the posterior end of the lower edge of the upper rib to divide the costo-transverse ligament. This allows the upper rib to hinge upwards more freely.

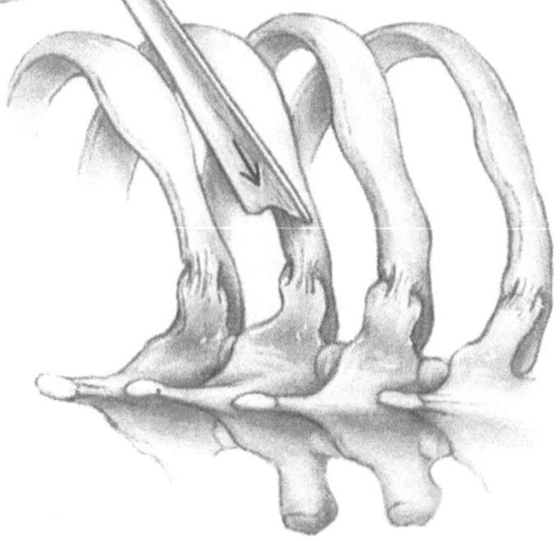

12b

12b Line of insertion of Semb chisel.

12c

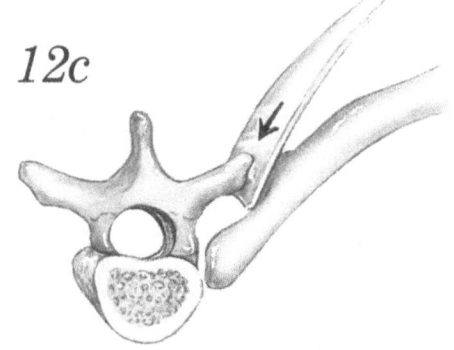

12c Division of the costo-transverse ligament.

13

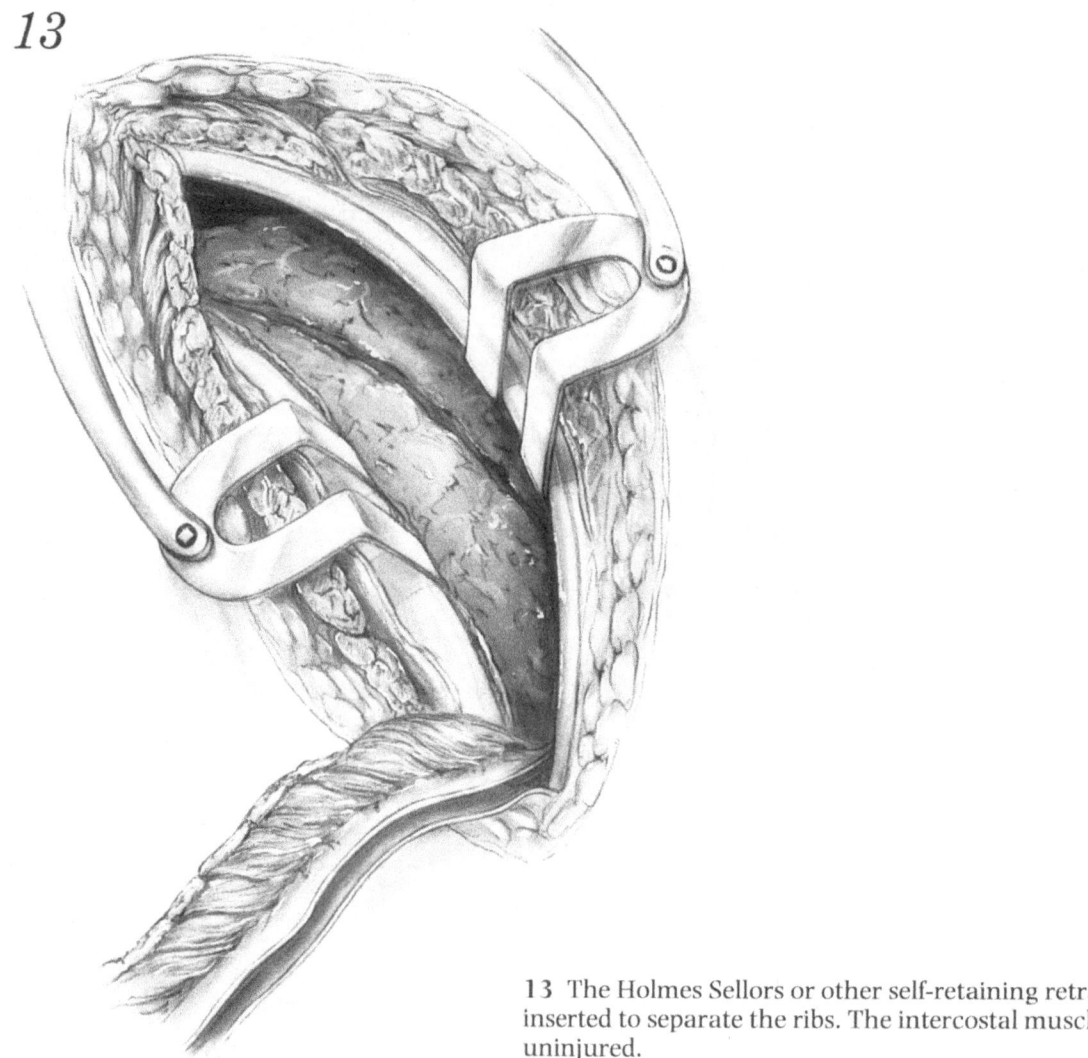

13 The Holmes Sellors or other self-retaining retractor is inserted to separate the ribs. The intercostal muscle bundle is uninjured.

Closure

14

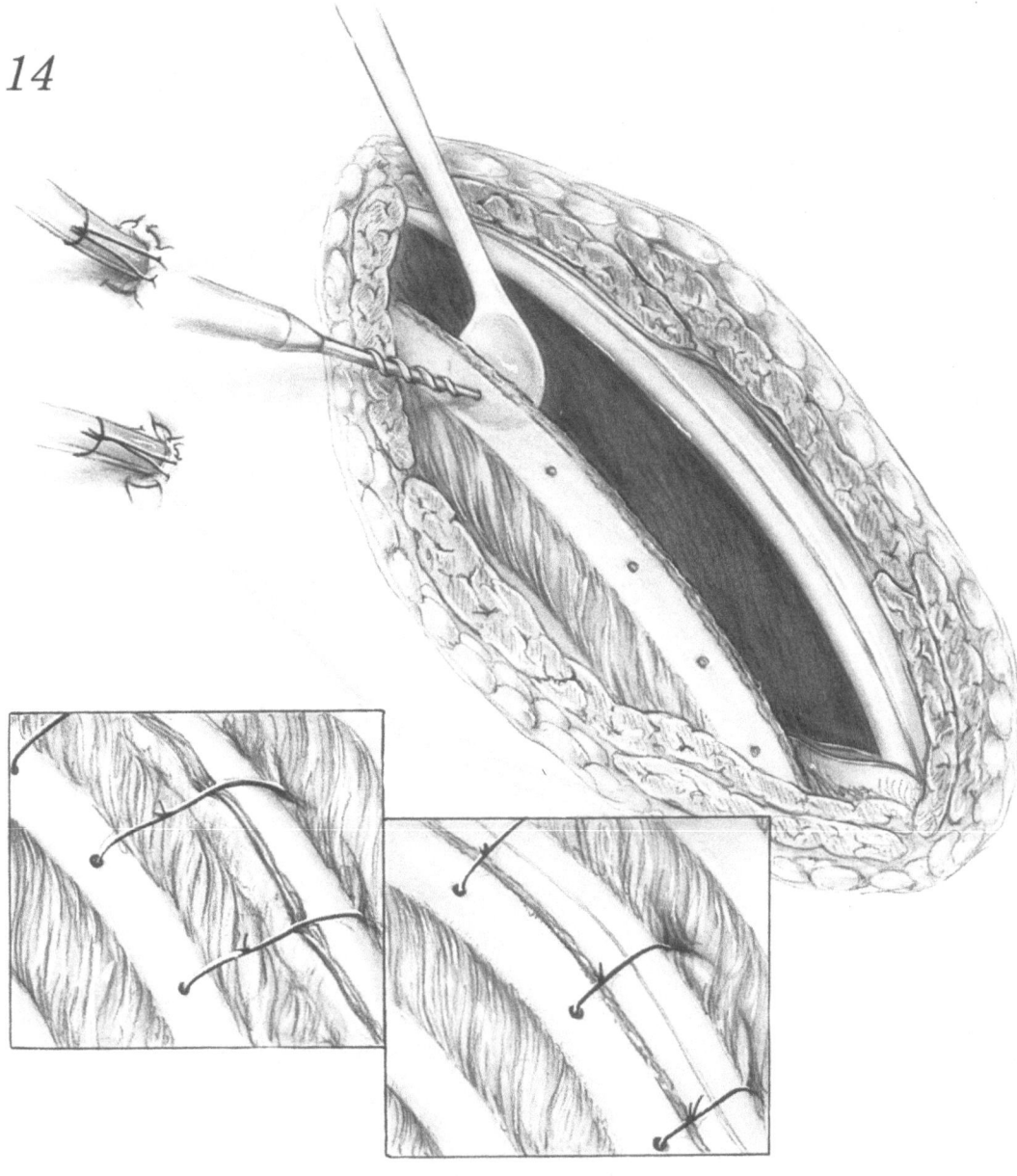

14 A chest drain is inserted through a separate stab incision. If an intercostal muscle bundle has been used then drill holes are made in the lower rib and the bare rib edges are approximated as shown. If the intercostal muscle bundle has not been used, then it is replaced.

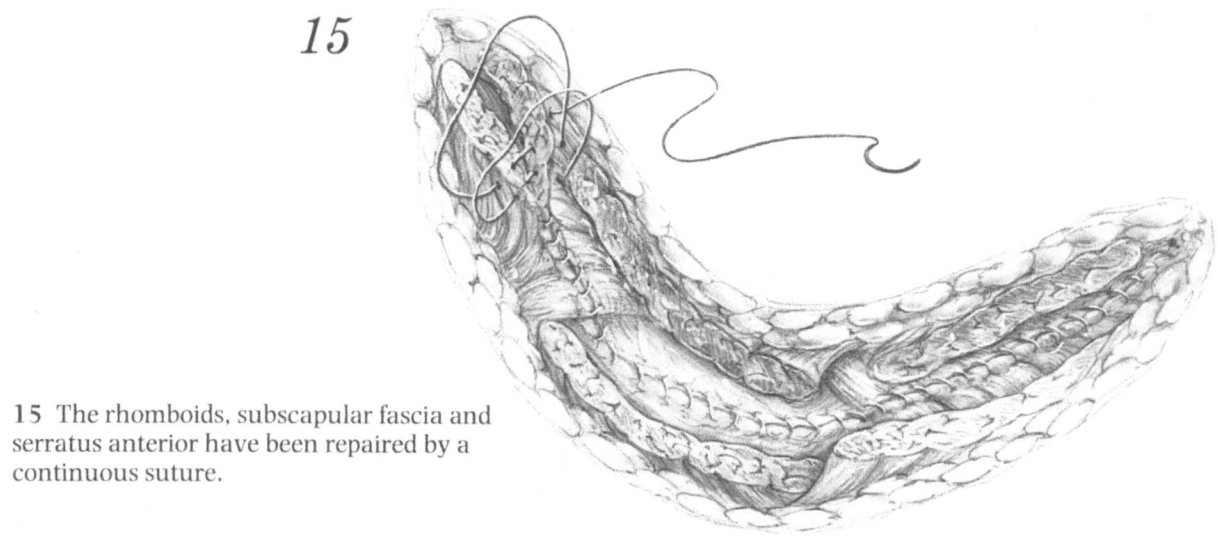

15 The rhomboids, subscapular fascia and serratus anterior have been repaired by a continuous suture.

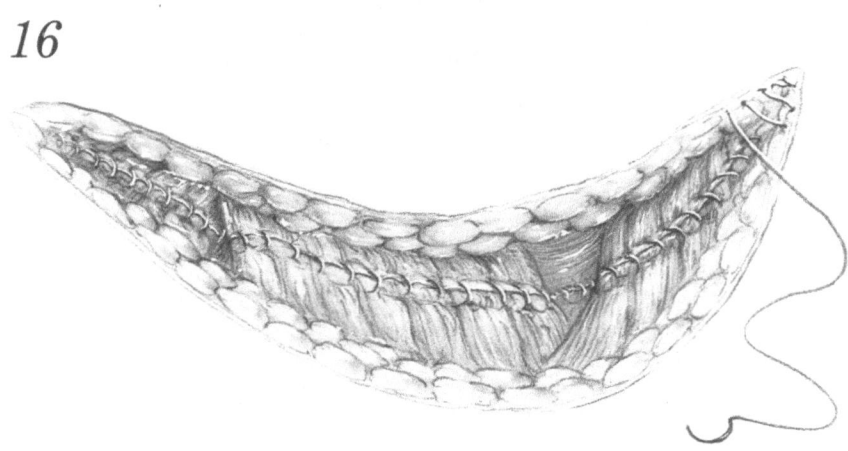

16 The trapezius and latissimus dorsi are next repaired by continuous suture. The subcutaneous layers and skin are closed routinely.

The patient should be transferred from the theatre with the chest drain unclamped but connected routinely to the underwater seal system. Care should be taken during manipulation to ensure that the chest drain is not dislodged or kinked.

Pain relief following thoracotomy may be facilitated by intra-operative application of the cryoprobe to the intercostal nerves over several dermatomes. Intravenous infusions of pethidine allow variation of analgesia for individual needs and during provocative manoeuvres such as physiotherapy.

The wound heals well since the muscles of the chest wall have a good blood supply. Care should be taken, however, to obtain early and complete mobility of the shoulder. There is often some erythema of the posterior and superior part of the incision, presumably related to the thicker skin over the back and the pressure borne by this area.

4 Right Thoracotomy

Right thoractomy provides adequate access for operation on the right lung and the right side of the posterior mediastinum. Anterior mediastinal masses with marked asymmetry to the right may also be approached through this incision. By division of the azygos arch this approach gives excellent exposure of the whole of the intrathoracic oesophagus and trachea and is the route of choice when approaching the main carina and the lower trachea.

Individual surgeons may vary the precise position of the incision, but they have in common the division of extra-thoracic muscles to mobilise the scapula and hence expose the thoracic cage. The muscle division is undertaken as low as possible so as to denervate as little of the extra-thoracic muscles as possible.

1

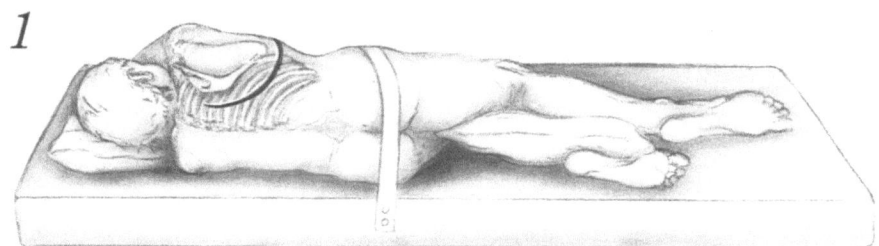

1 The incision in relation to the scapula and ribs is shown from the back. The posterior superior limit of the incision for a standard posterolateral thoractomy extends to midway between the thoracic spinous processes and the spine of the scapula.

2

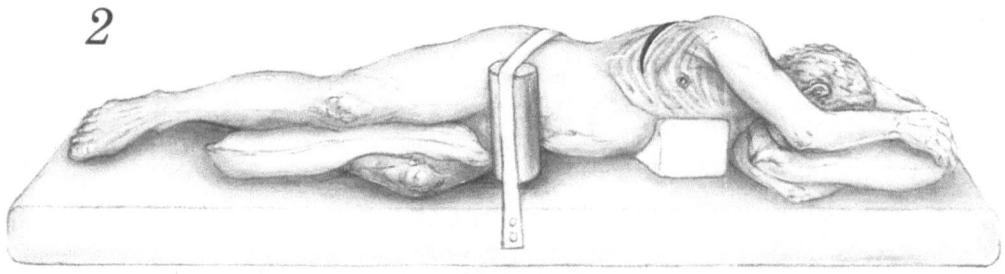

2 The anterior limit of the incision over the sixth or fifth costo-chondral junction.

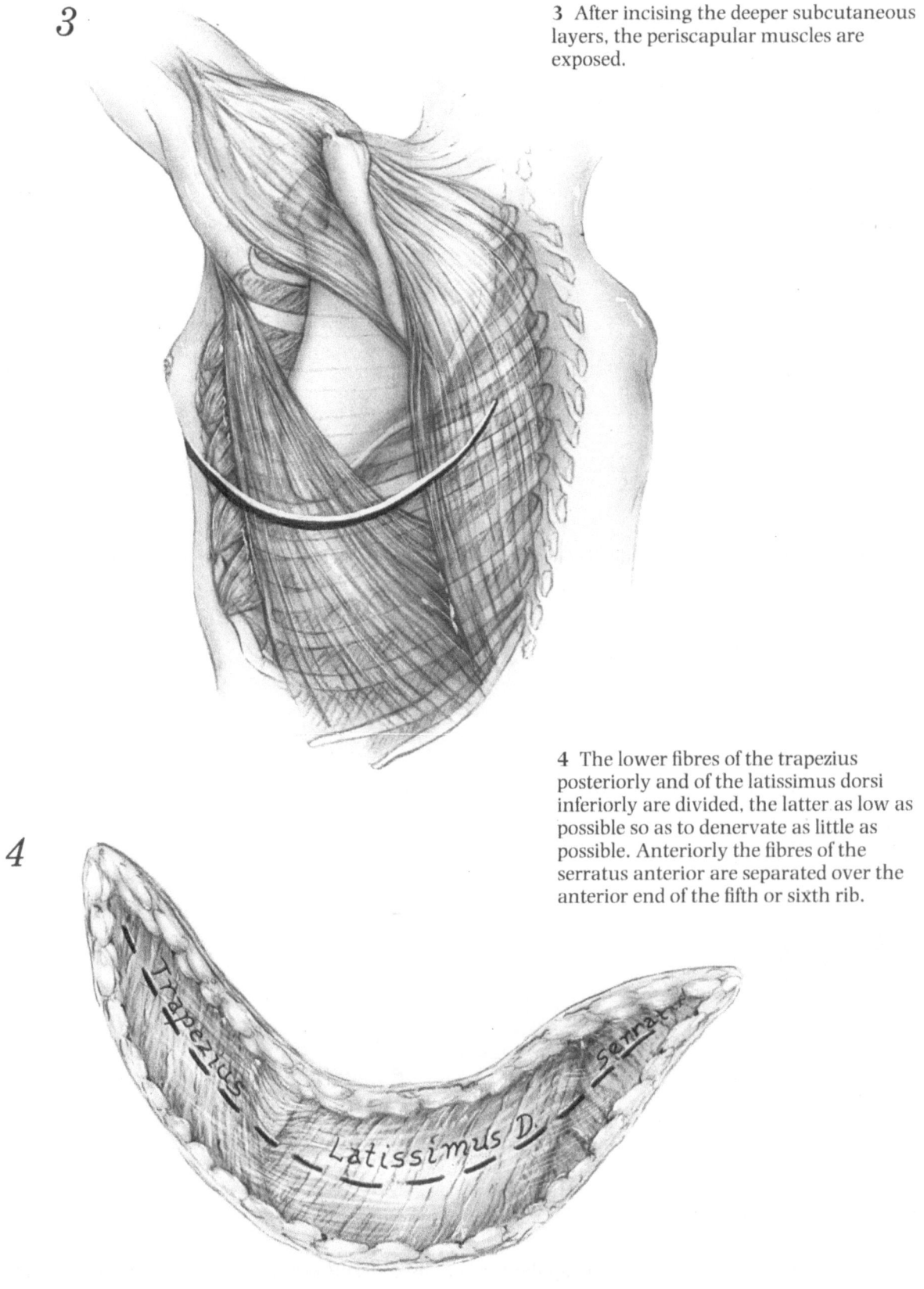

3 After incising the deeper subcutaneous layers, the periscapular muscles are exposed.

4 The lower fibres of the trapezius posteriorly and of the latissimus dorsi inferiorly are divided, the latter as low as possible so as to denervate as little as possible. Anteriorly the fibres of the serratus anterior are separated over the anterior end of the fifth or sixth rib.

5

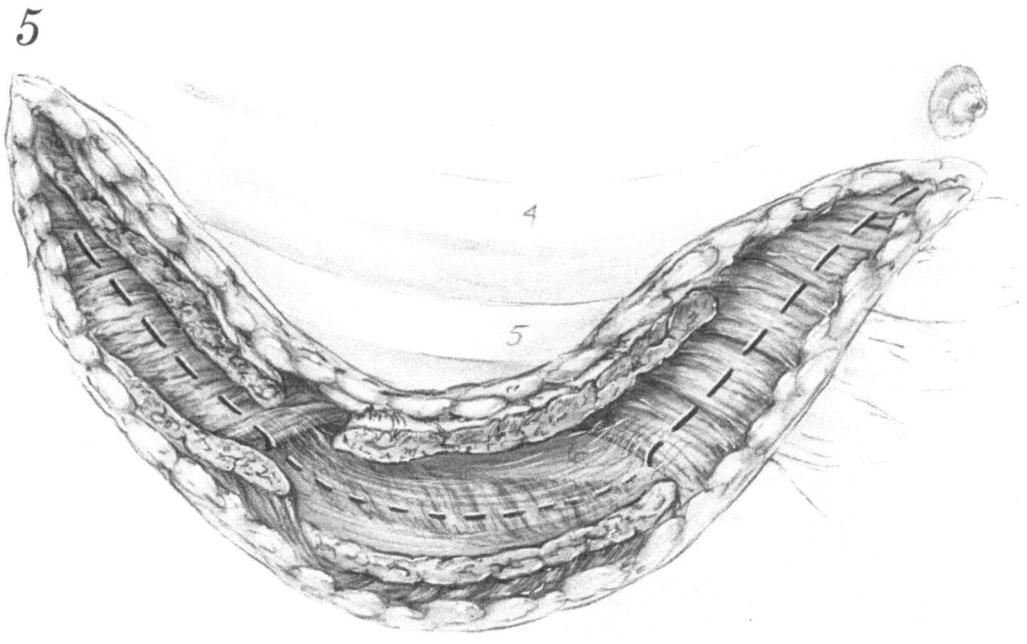

5 Posteriorly the rhomboids are divided in the same plane as the serratus anterior in front.

6

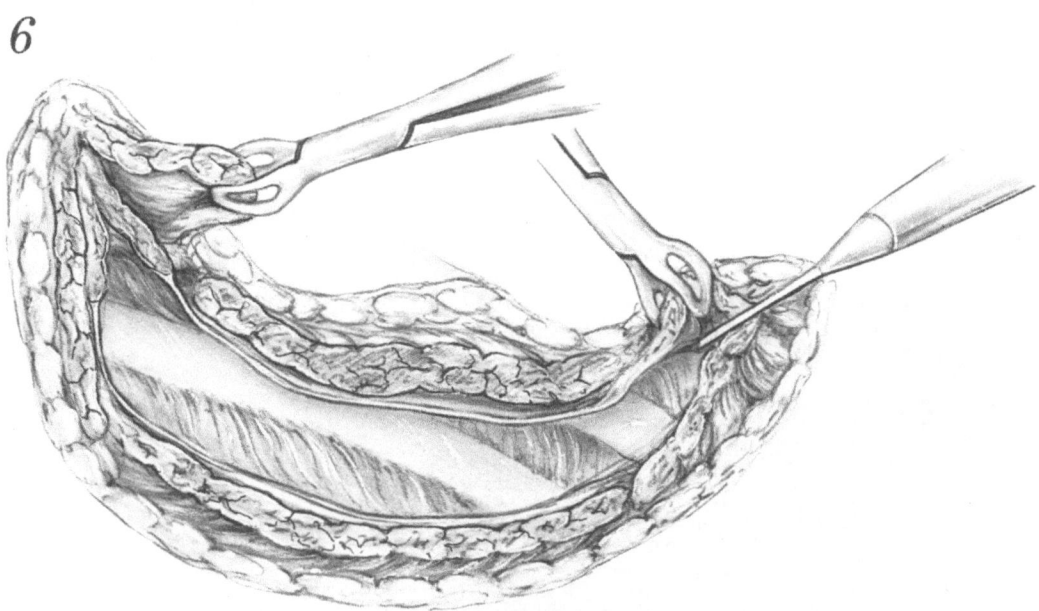

6 Between these two muscles the subscapular fascia is dissected off so as to interfere as little as possible with post-operative movement of the scapula.

7

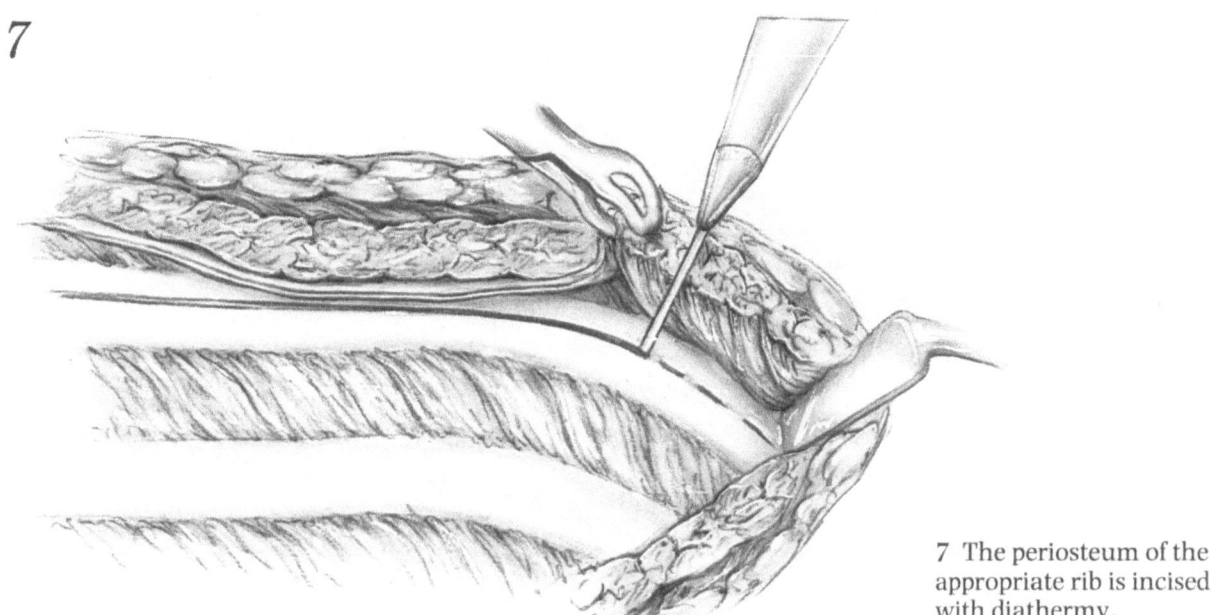

7 The periosteum of the appropriate rib is incised with diathermy.

8a

8a The lower half of the periosteum is elevated anteriorly with the rugine sufficiently to allow the insertion of the blade of the rugine. Note that the intercostal muscles are not incised.

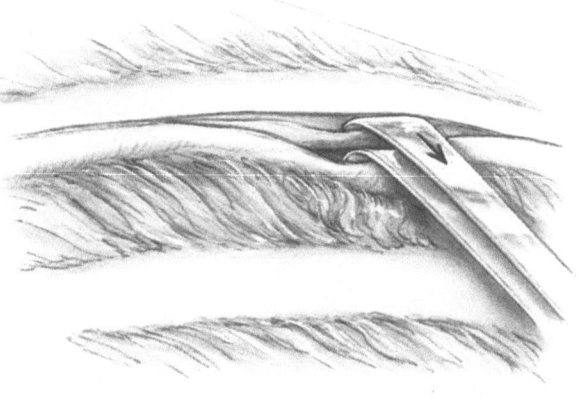

8b

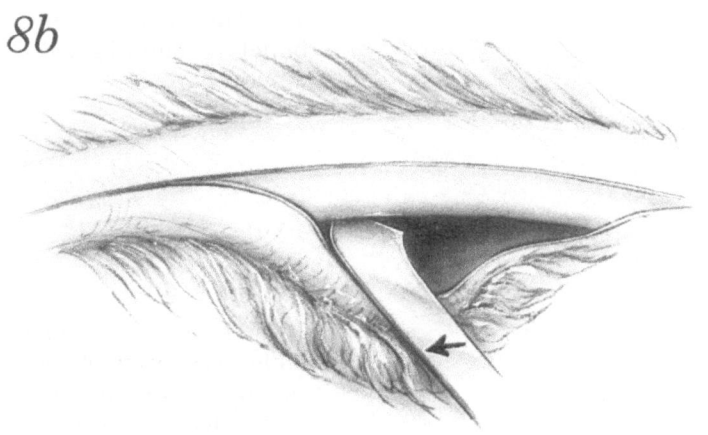

8b The rugine is used to strip the periosteum off the lower border of the rib, as shown from front to back.

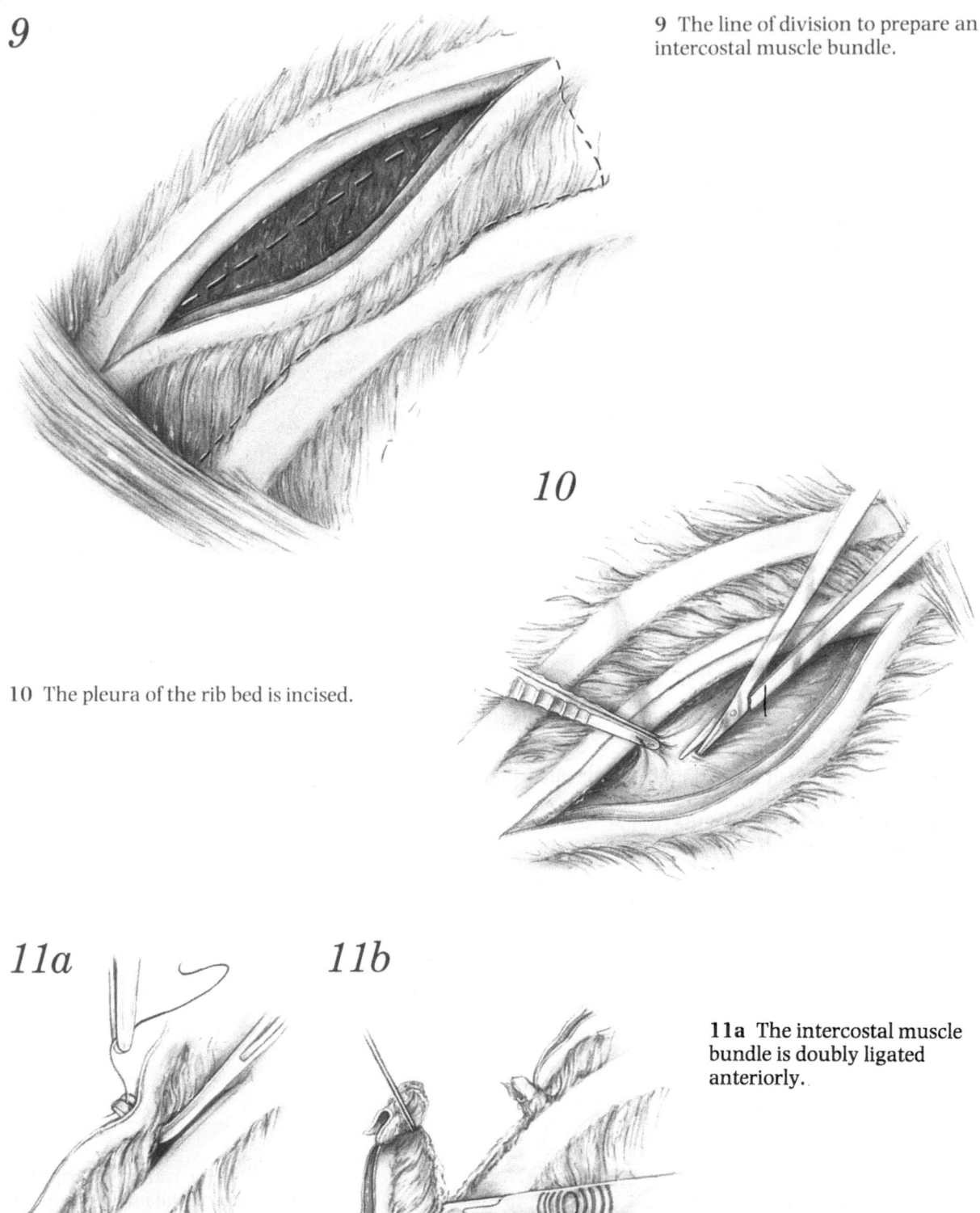

9 The line of division to prepare an intercostal muscle bundle.

10 The pleura of the rib bed is incised.

11a The intercostal muscle bundle is doubly ligated anteriorly.

11b The intercostal muscle bundle is now cut off the superior edge of the lower rib as far back as possible.

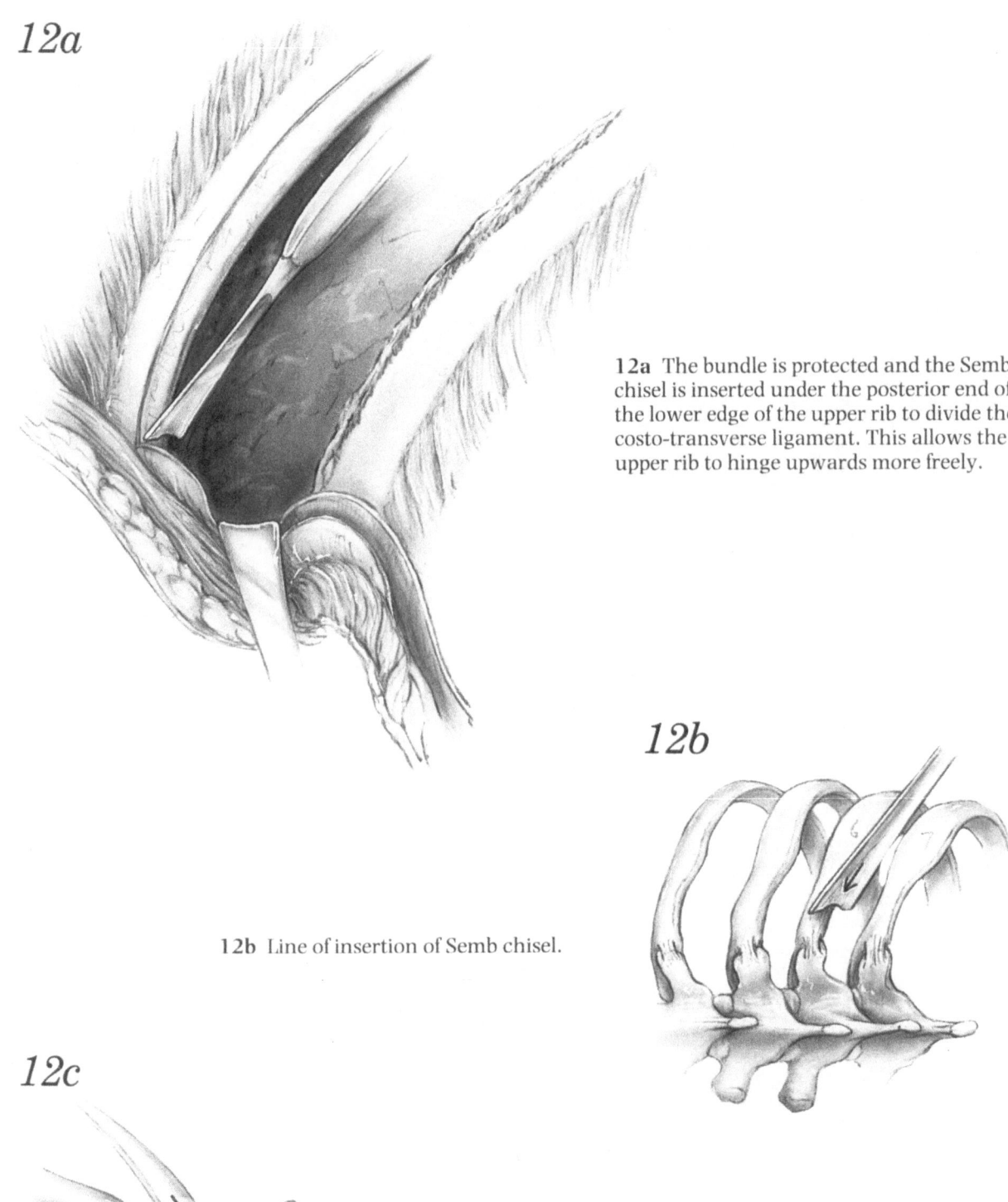

12a

12a The bundle is protected and the Semb chisel is inserted under the posterior end of the lower edge of the upper rib to divide the costo-transverse ligament. This allows the upper rib to hinge upwards more freely.

12b

12b Line of insertion of Semb chisel.

12c

12c Division of costo-transverse ligament.

13

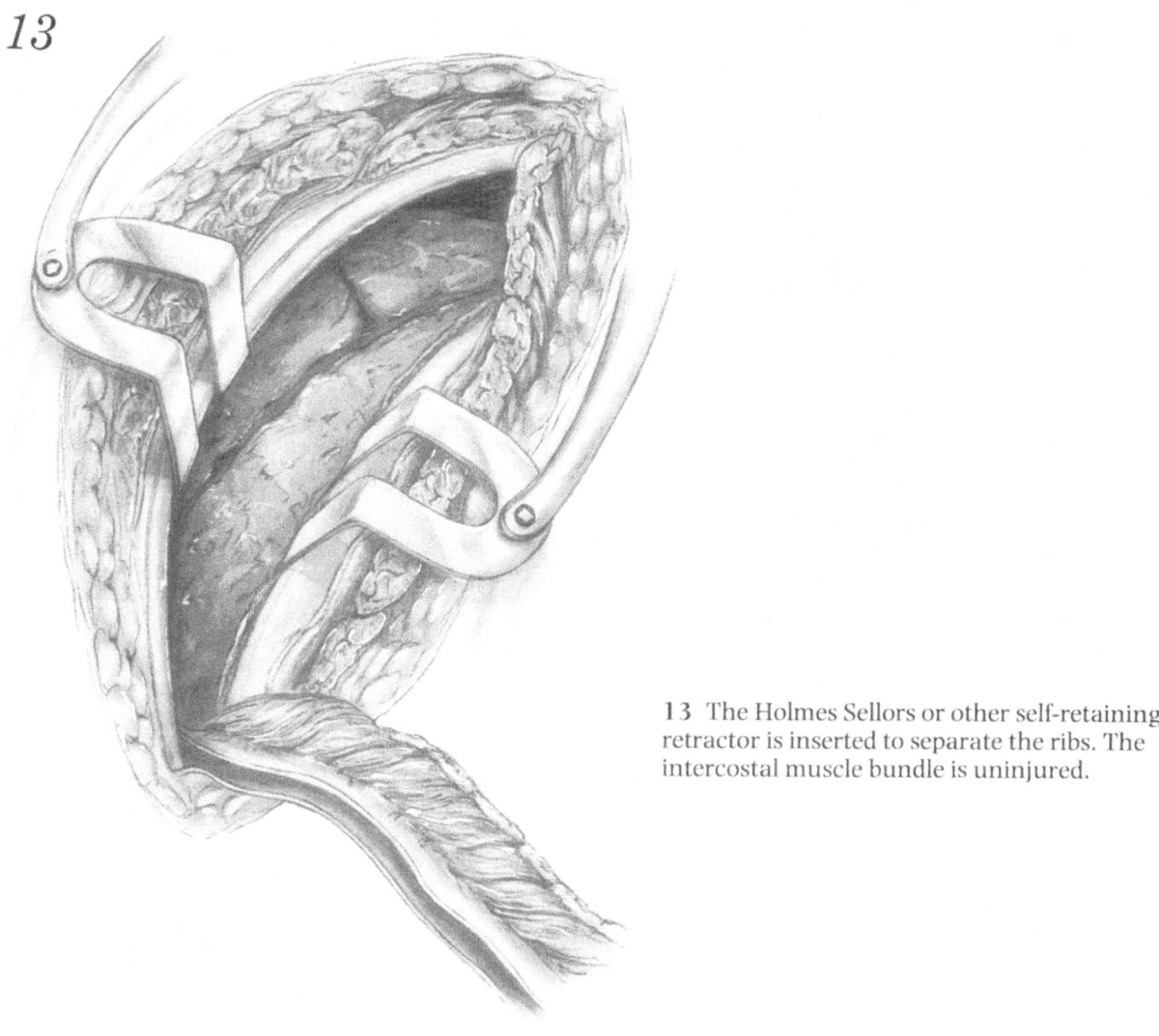

13 The Holmes Sellors or other self-retaining retractor is inserted to separate the ribs. The intercostal muscle bundle is uninjured.

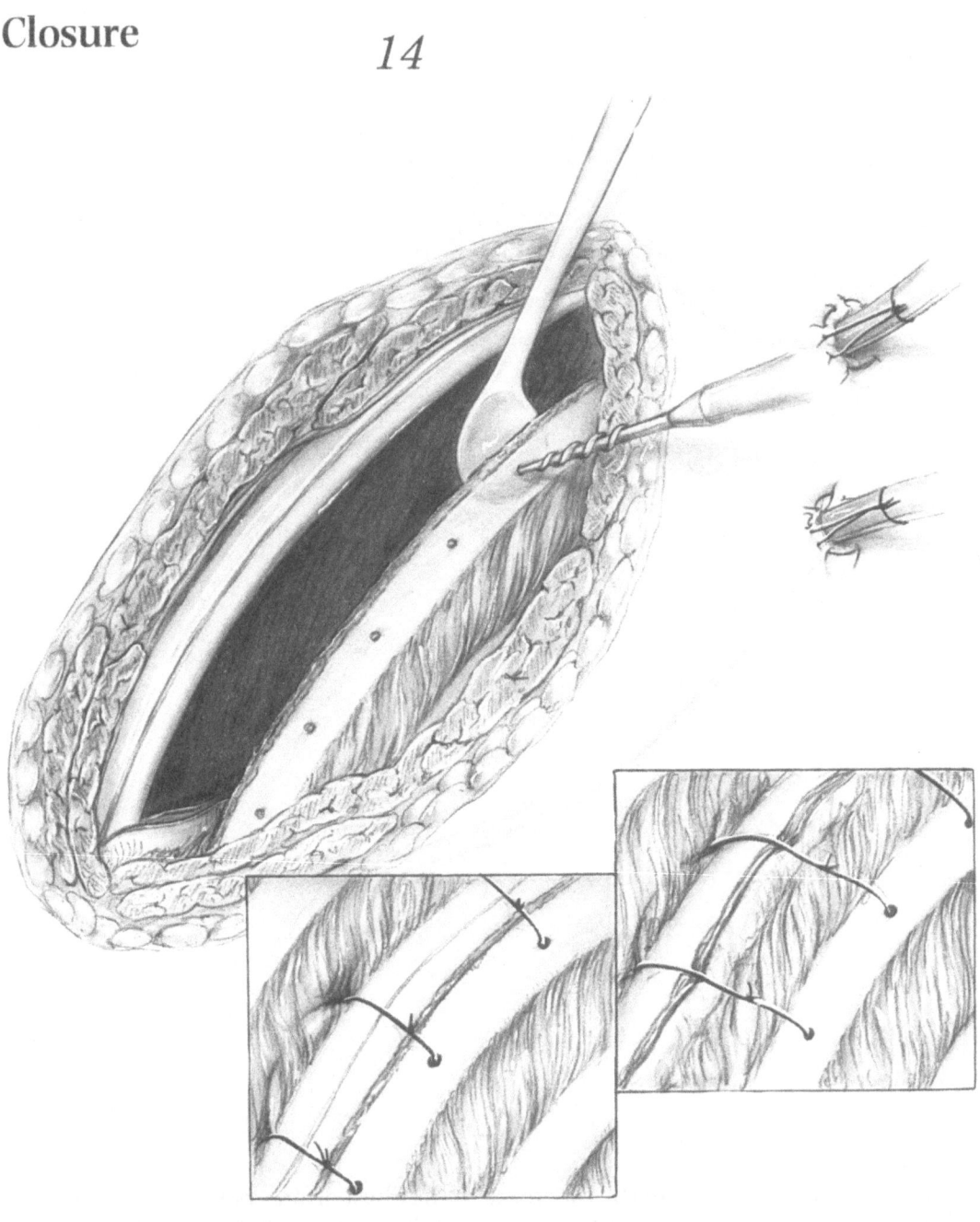

14 A chest drain is inserted through a separate stab incision. If an intercostal muscle bundle has been used then drill holes are made in the lower rib and the bare rib edges are approximated as shown. If the intercostal muscle bundle has not been used, then it is replaced.

15

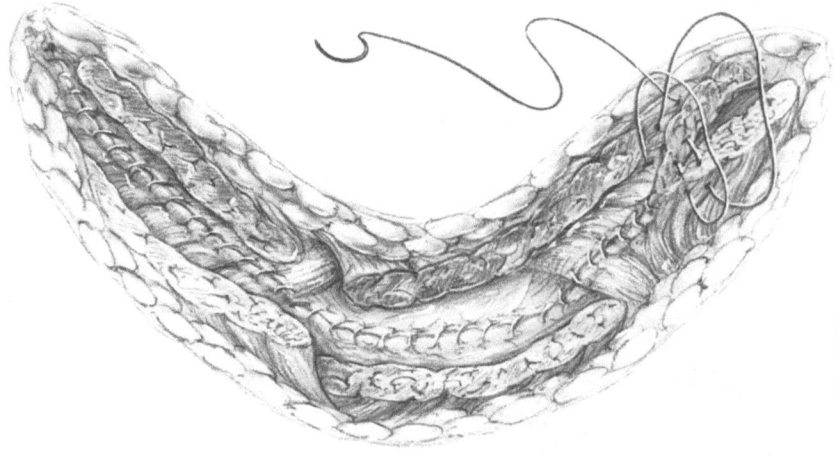

15 The rhomboids, subscapular fascia and serratus anterior have been repaired by a continuous suture.

16

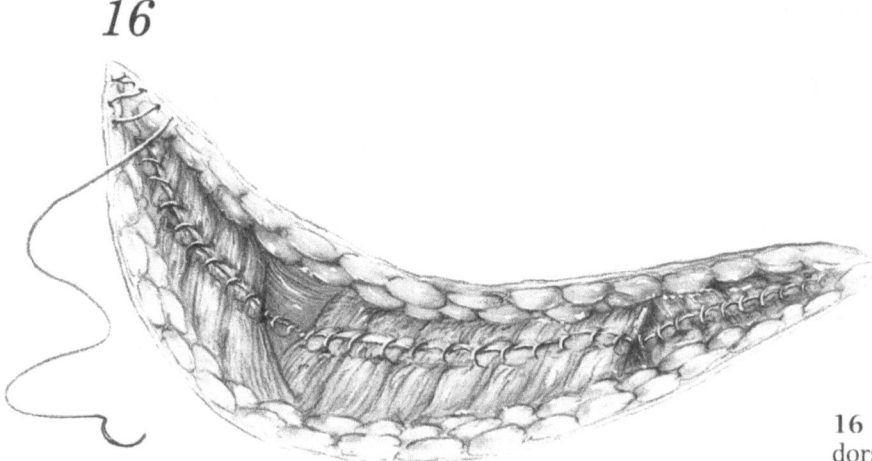

16 The trapezius and latissimus dorsi are next repaired by continuous suture. The subcutaneous layers and skin are closed routinely.

The patient should be transferred from the theatre with the chest drain unclamped but connected routinely to the underwater seal system. Care should be taken during all manipulations to ensure that the chest drain is not dislodged or kinked.

Pain relief following thoracotomy may be facilitated by intra-operative application of the cryoprobe to the intercostal nerves over several dermatomes. Intravenous infusions of pethidine allow variation of analgesia for individual needs and during provocative manoeuvres such as physiotherapy.

The wound heals well since the muscles of the chest wall have a good blood supply. Care should be taken, however, to obtain early and complete mobility of the shoulder. There is often some erythema of the posterior and superior part of the incision, presumably related to the thicker skin over the back and the pressure borne by this area.

5 Right Upper Lobectomy

Right upper lobectomy is indicated whenever the disease process is limited to the right upper lobe. The commonest such indication in the western world is carcinoma of the bronchus. The tumour and involved lymph nodes must be confined to the lobe, and lines of resection through vessels and bronchus should be clear of tumour. When undertaken for pulmonary sepsis, pre-operative physiotherapy may produce a temporary but important improvement in the patient's condition and help minimise post-operative sputum difficulties. All patients should be instructed pre-operatively in the physiotherapy manoeuvres which will be undertaken post-operatively. Prophylactic antibiotics started with the premedication and continued for 24 h have been shown to reduce the incidence of wound infection, but will have no influence on the more serious problems of chest infection and infection of the pleural space.

An endobronchial tube passed by the anaesthetist will allow single lung ventilation. The collapse of the lung on the side of surgery will minimise the competing aims of surgeon and anaesthetist.

1

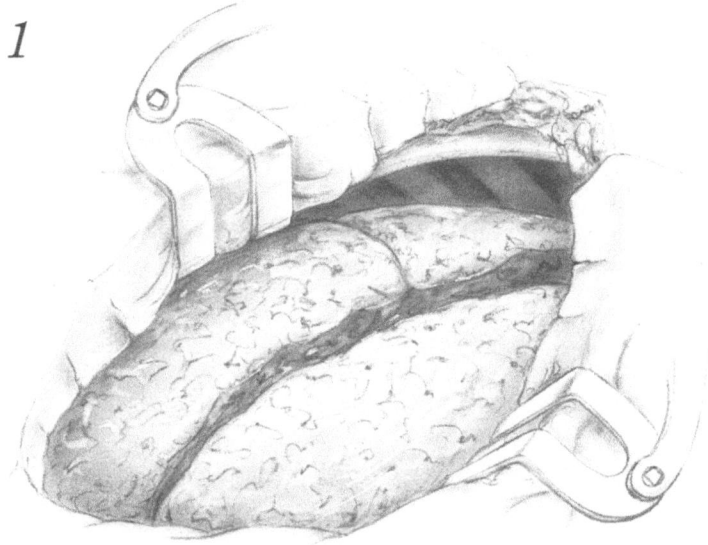

1 The chest has been opened by stripping the lower border of the fifth rib.

2

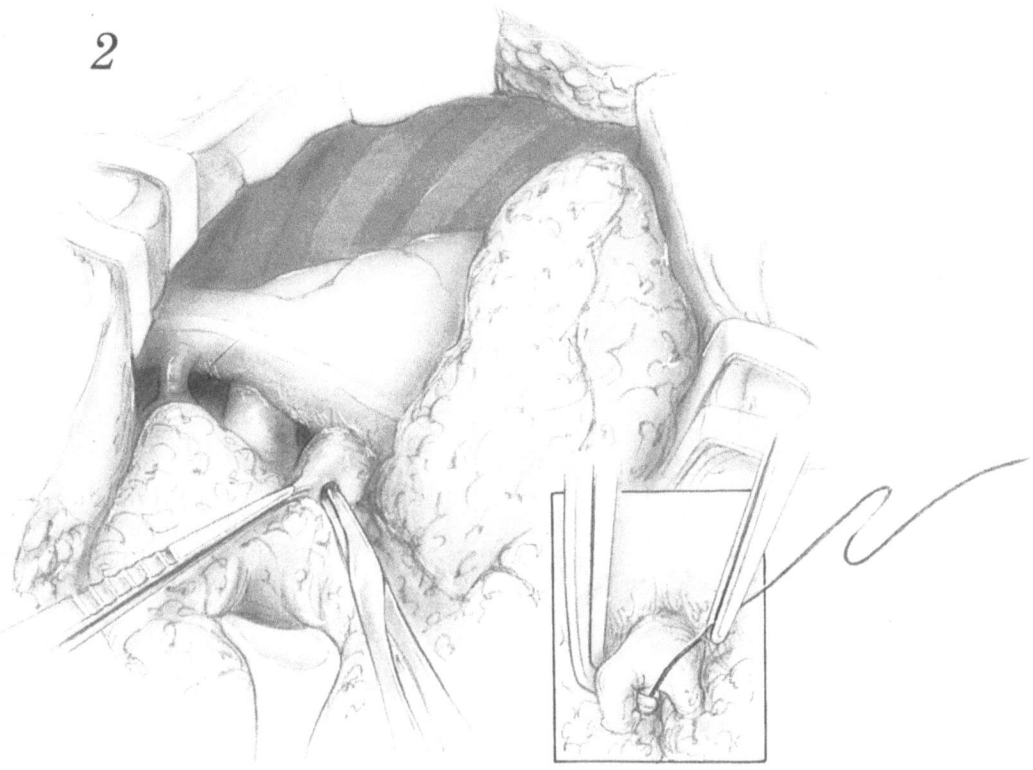

2 The right superior pulmonary vein has been exposed and dissected so as to identify its middle lobe tributary. The division draining the upper lobe is tied.

3

3 The azygos vein has been tied at its origin and termination and the superior vena cava is retracted forwards to expose the para-aortic fossa. The vagus has been divided below its recurrent branch and the lymph nodes have been dissected downwards towards the right pulmonary artery.

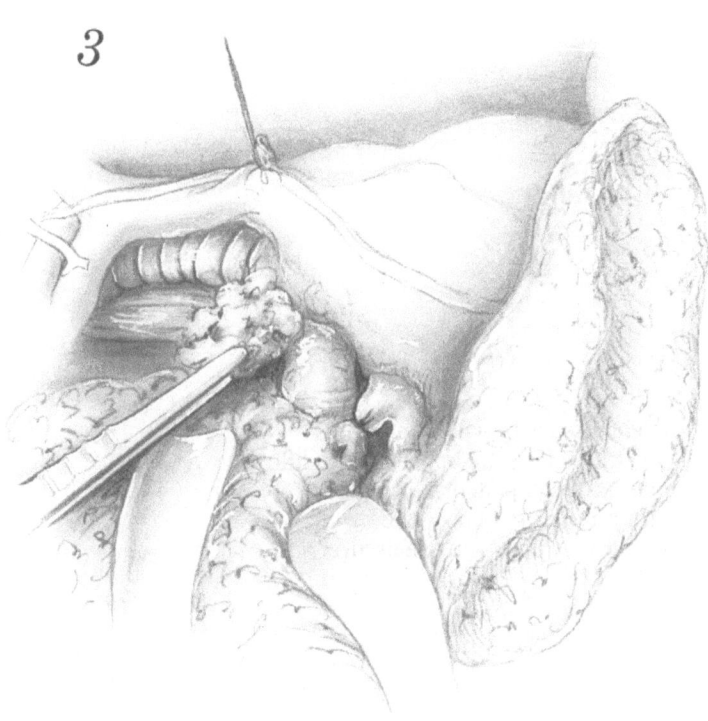

4

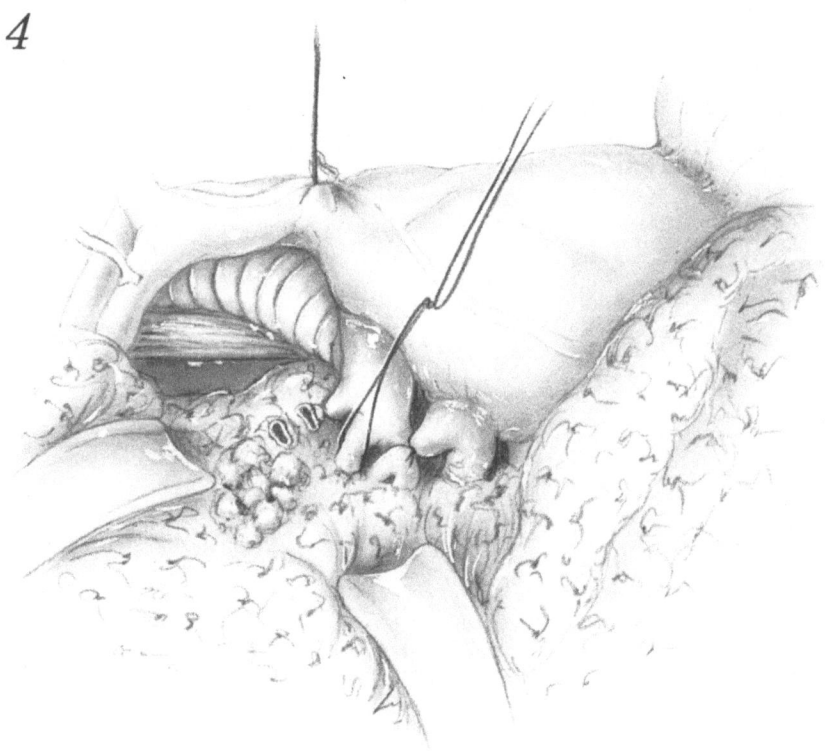

4 The branches of the pulmonary artery to the upper lobe are identified, tied and divided.

5

5 The fissure between the right lower lobe and the upper and middle lobes is developed, dissecting the lymph nodes to expose the pulmonary artery in the fissure.

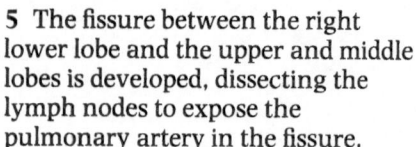

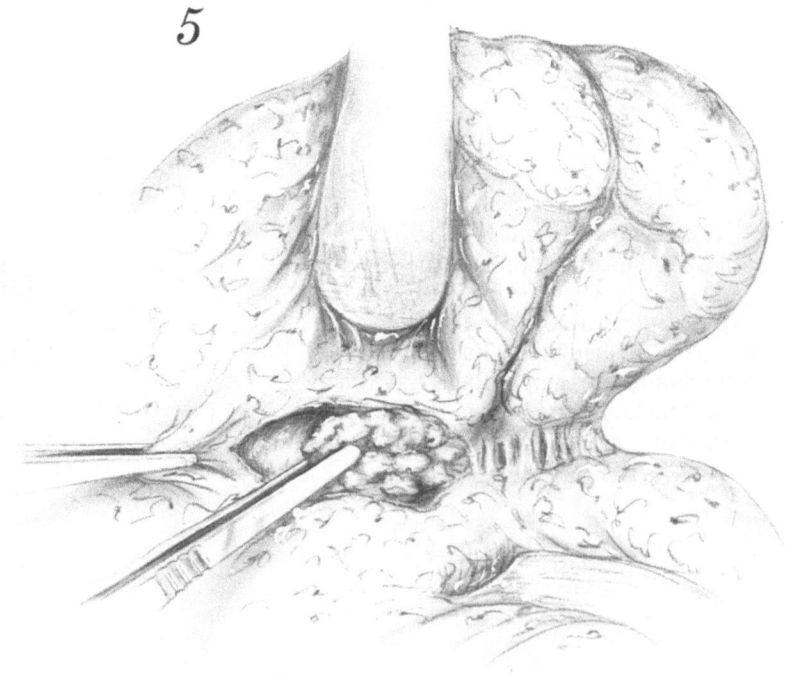

6 The fissure has been developed and the branches of the pulmonary artery in the fissure to the right upper lobe are identified and tied.

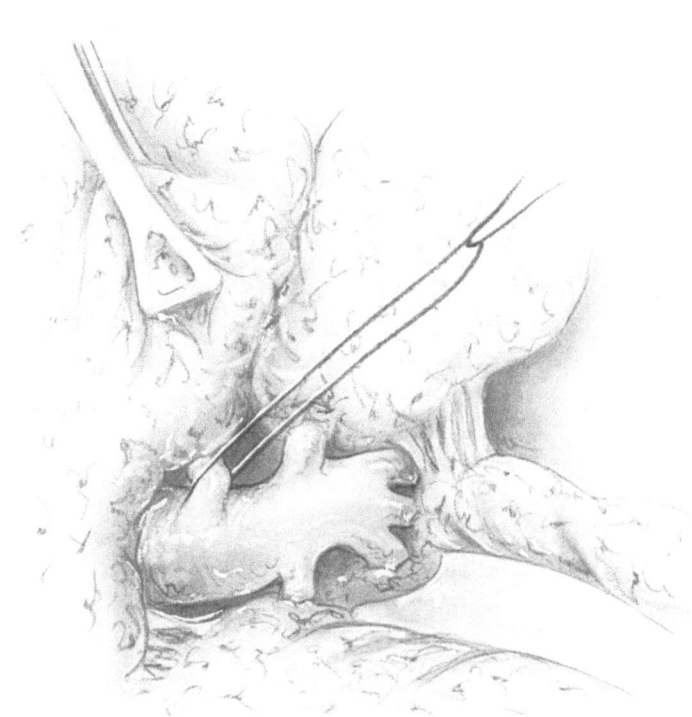

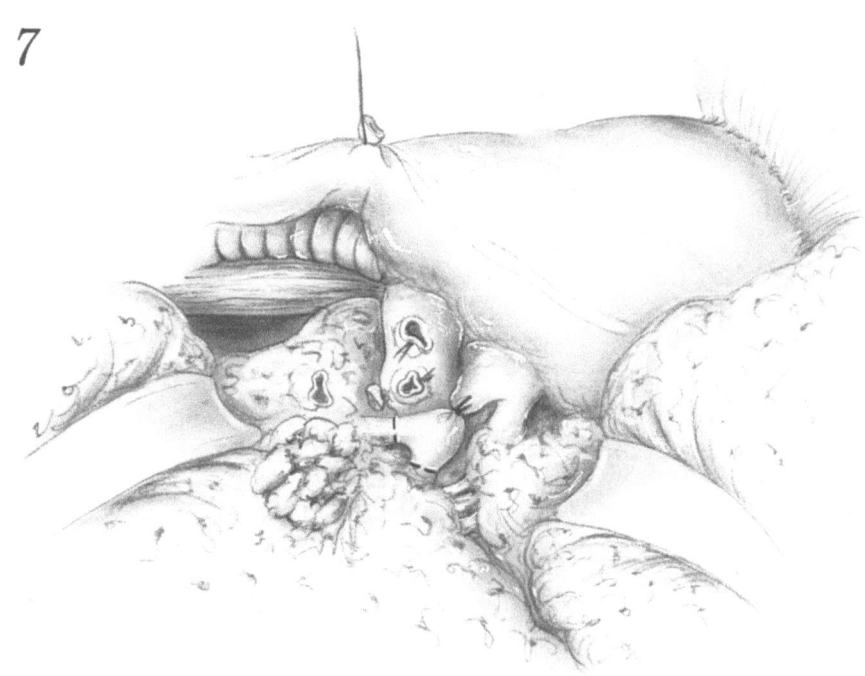

7 The right superior pulmonary vein is dissected to its tributaries, which are tied; the vein is then divided.

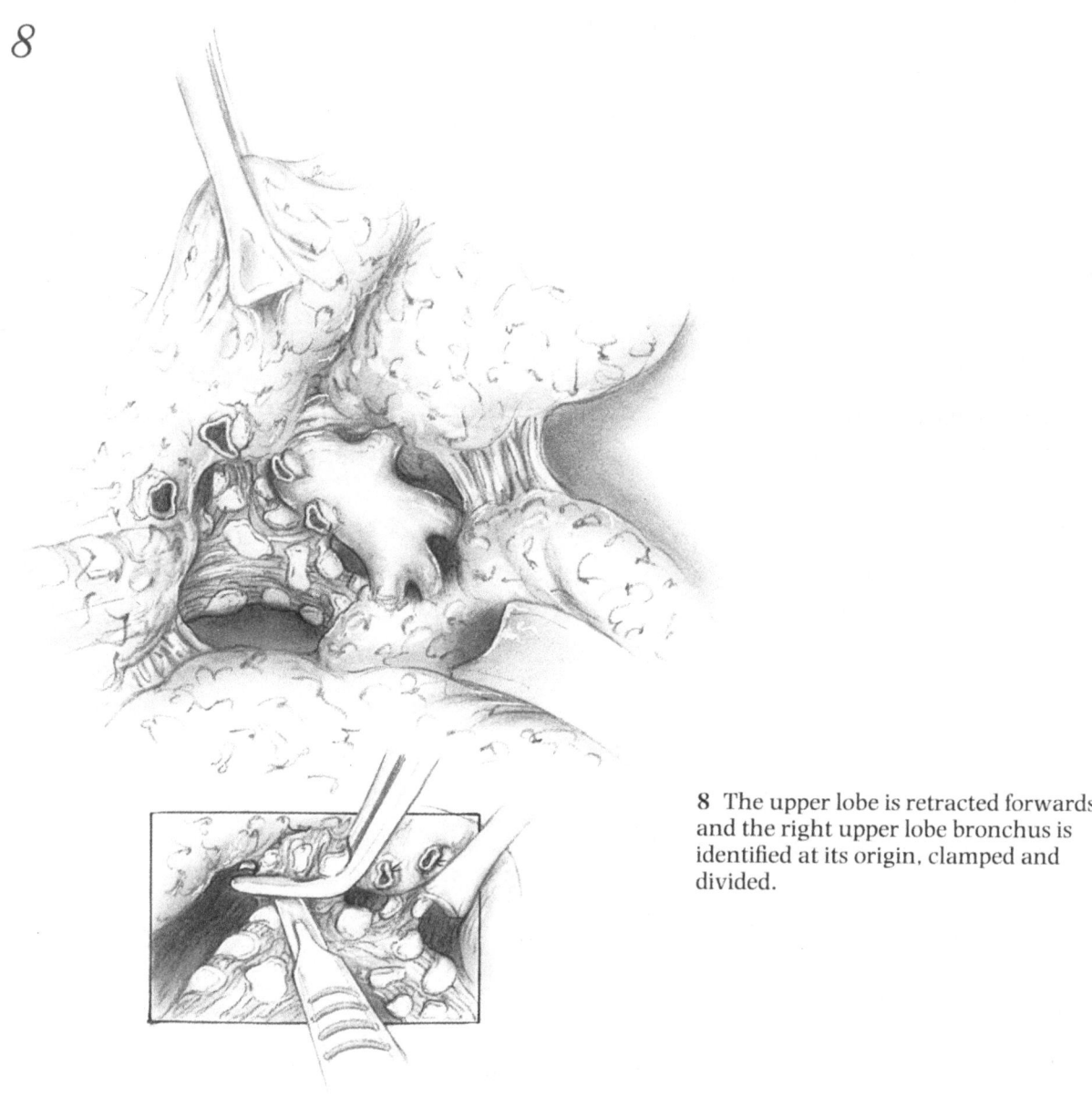

8 The upper lobe is retracted forwards and the right upper lobe bronchus is identified at its origin, clamped and divided.

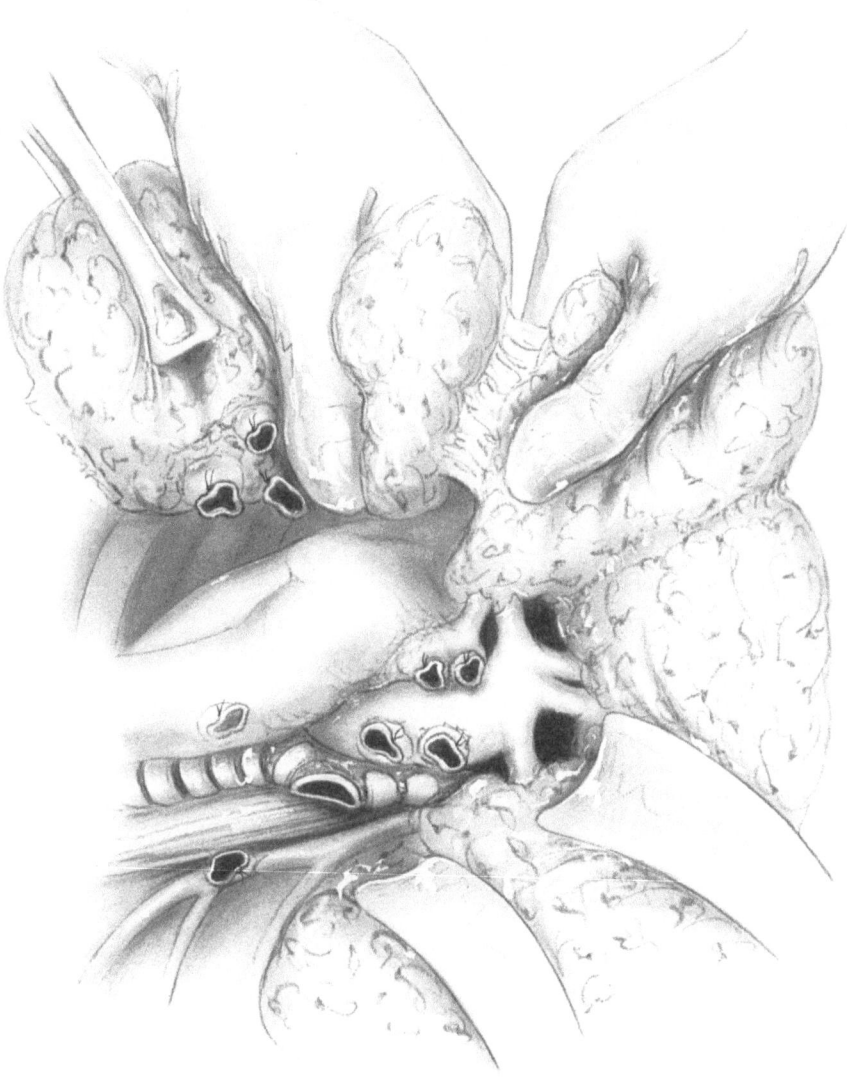

9 The upper lobe is finally separated from the middle lobe by blunt and sharp dissection and removed.

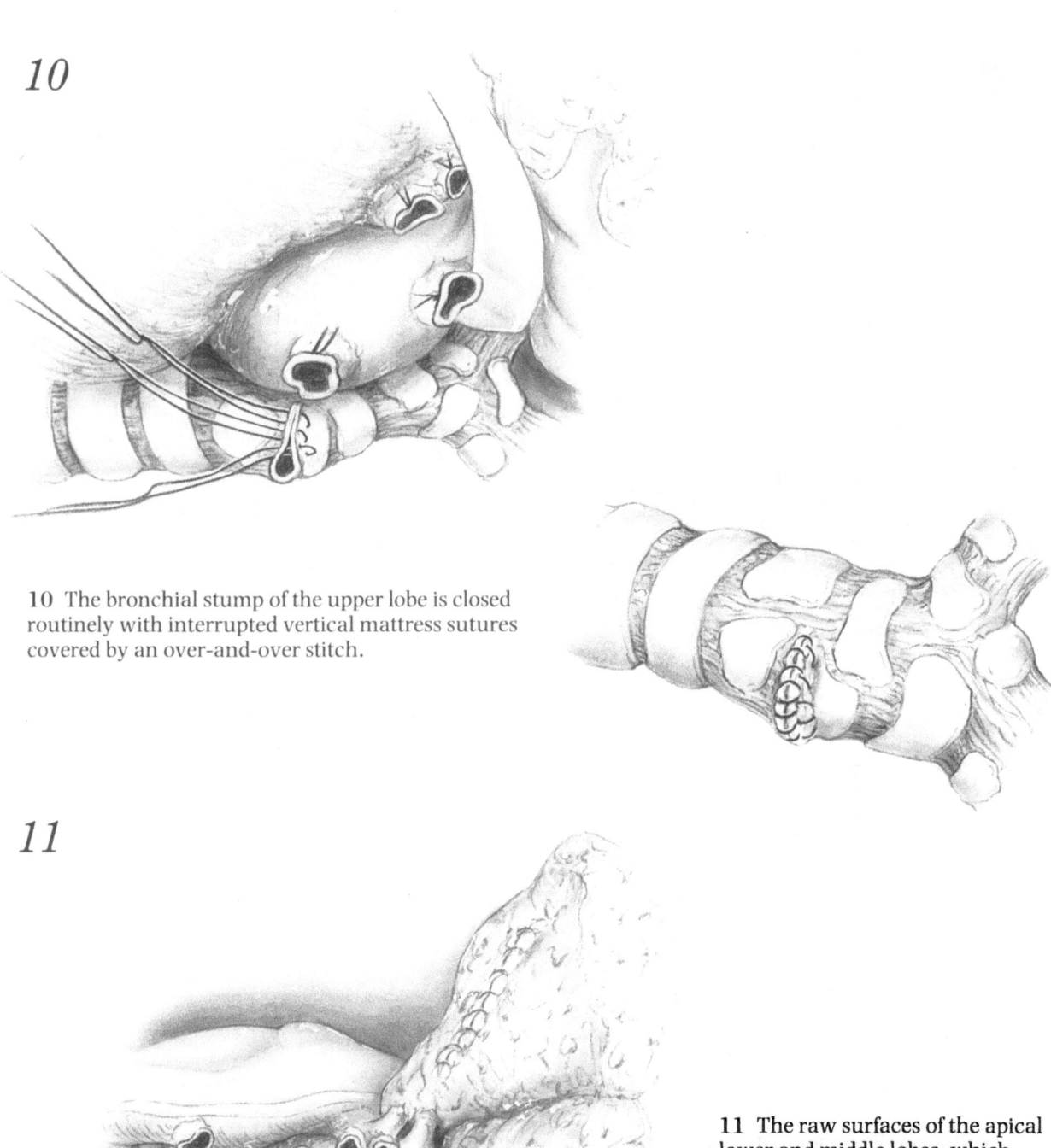

10

10 The bronchial stump of the upper lobe is closed routinely with interrupted vertical mattress sutures covered by an over-and-over stitch.

11

11 The raw surfaces of the apical lower and middle lobes, which may have resulted from an incomplete fissure, are oversewn with an absorbable suture in two layers. The chest is then closed routinely.

The incision is closed in layers with anterior and posterior drainage tubes, with sideholes, extending up to the apex. The chest drains should not be clamped during transport of the patient back to the ward and care must be taken that the drains are not dislodged or kinked during movement. Once the patient is back in the ward the chest drains are connected to suction which must have careful control and be capable of high volume suction. Suction should be sufficient to maintain a negative pressure resulting in continuous bubbling throughout the respiratory cycle. Tubes are removed sequentially when all drainage and air leak has stopped.

Prophylactic antibiotics should be discontinued after 24 h. Antibiotics are thereafter only indicated for specific infective problems.

Adequate pain relief should be ensured to permit early and full movement of the shoulder and to allow the patient to co-operate with the physiotherapist in expectoration. Sputum problems are common following pulmonary resection, and if not dealt with promptly, will lead to life-threatening complications such as pulmonary infection. If sputum retention occurs despite adequate analgesia and intensive physiotherapy, suction bronchoscopy may be necessary. The insertion of a minitracheostomy tube through the cricothyroid membrane has largely replaced the performance of formal tracheostomy.

Cardiac dysrhythmias, particularly atrial tachycardias, are common following pulmonary resection and prophylactic digoxin is often used in the elderly.

With the emphasis on early mobilisation, deep venous thrombosis and pulmonary embolism are now rarities and there is no evidence that low dose heparin is of any value.

6 Right Lower Lobectomy

Right lower lobectomy is indicated whenever the disease process is limited to the right lower lobe. The commonest such indication in the western world is carcinoma of the bronchus. The tumour and involved lymph nodes must be confined to the lobe, and lines of resection through vessels and bronchus should be clear of tumour. When undertaken for pulmonary sepsis, pre-operative physiotherapy may produce a temporary but important improvement in the patient's condition and help minimise post-operative sputum difficulties. All patients should be instructed pre-operatively in the physiotherapy manoeuvres which will be undertaken post-operatively. Prophylactic antibiotics commenced with the premedication and continued for 24 h have been shown to reduce the incidence of wound infection but will have no influence on the more serious problems of chest infection and infection of the pleural space.

An endobronchial tube passed by the anaesthetist will allow single lung ventilation. The collapse of the lung on the side of surgery will minimise the competing aims of surgeon and anaesthetist.

1

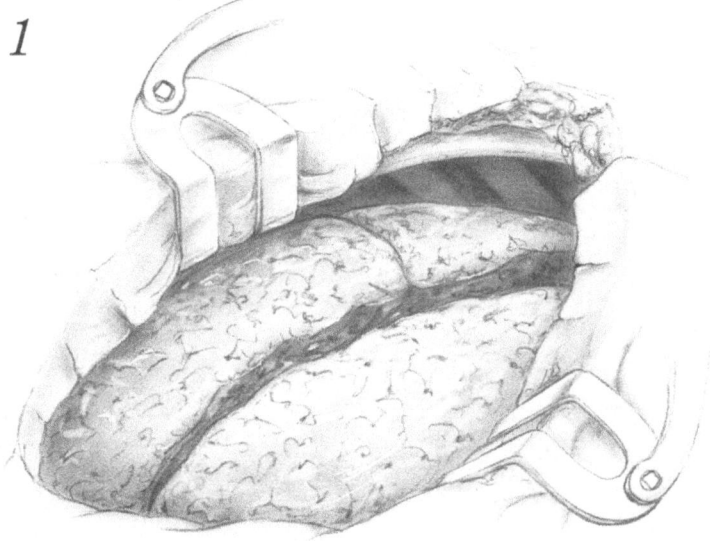

1 The chest has been entered by stripping the lower border of the fifth or sixth rib.

2

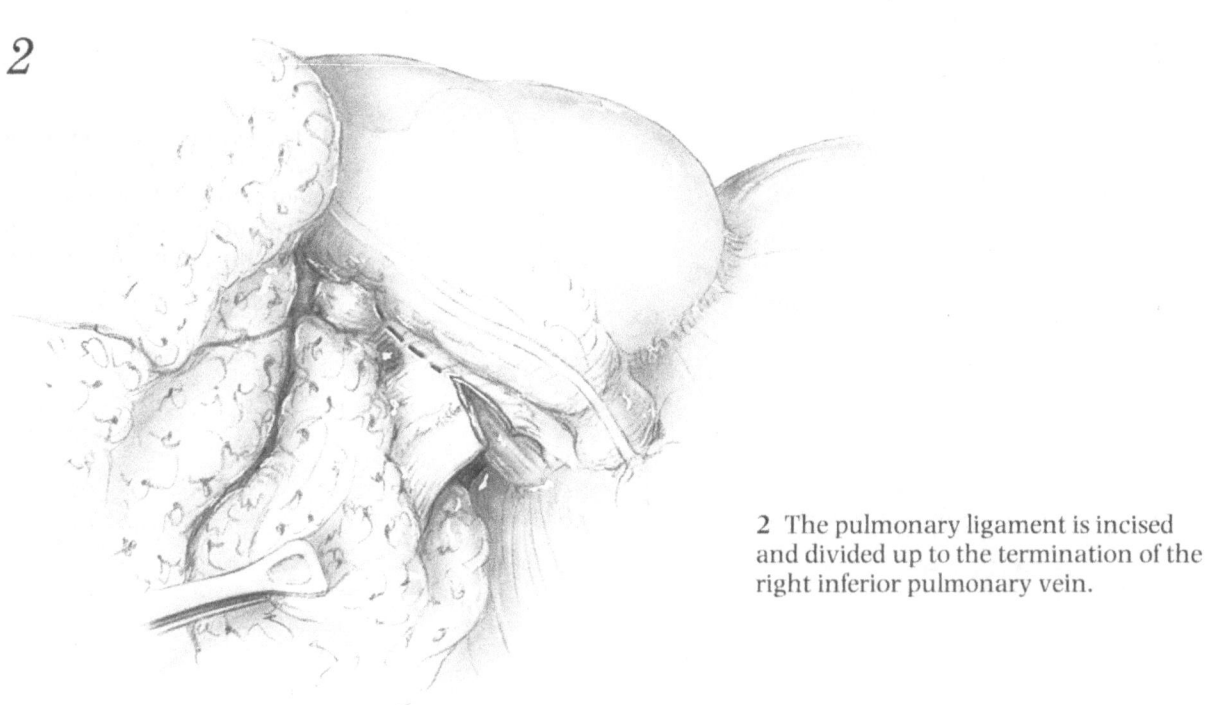

2 The pulmonary ligament is incised and divided up to the termination of the right inferior pulmonary vein.

3

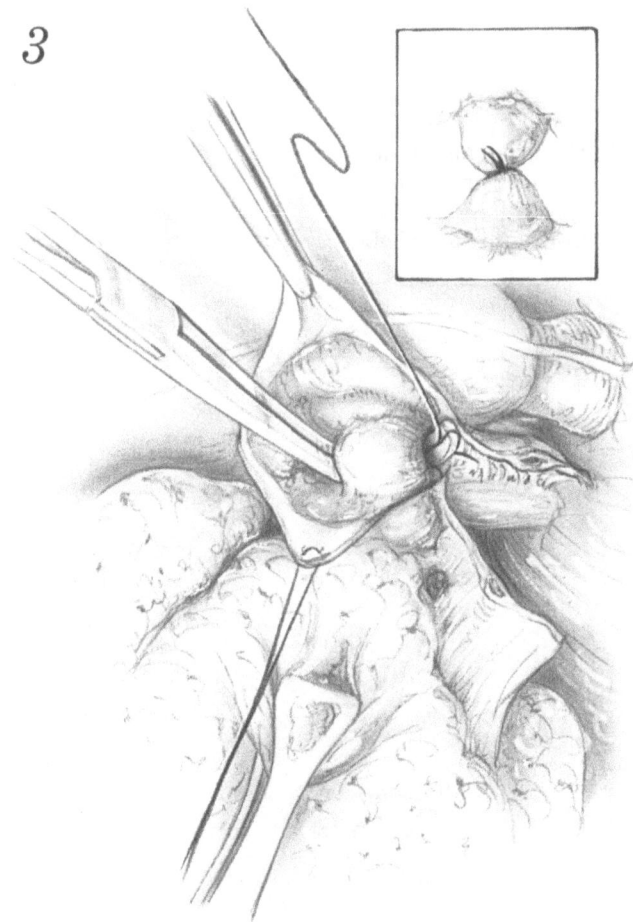

3 The pericardium has been opened to expose the termination of the right inferior pulmonary vein, and this is tied as a first step.

4

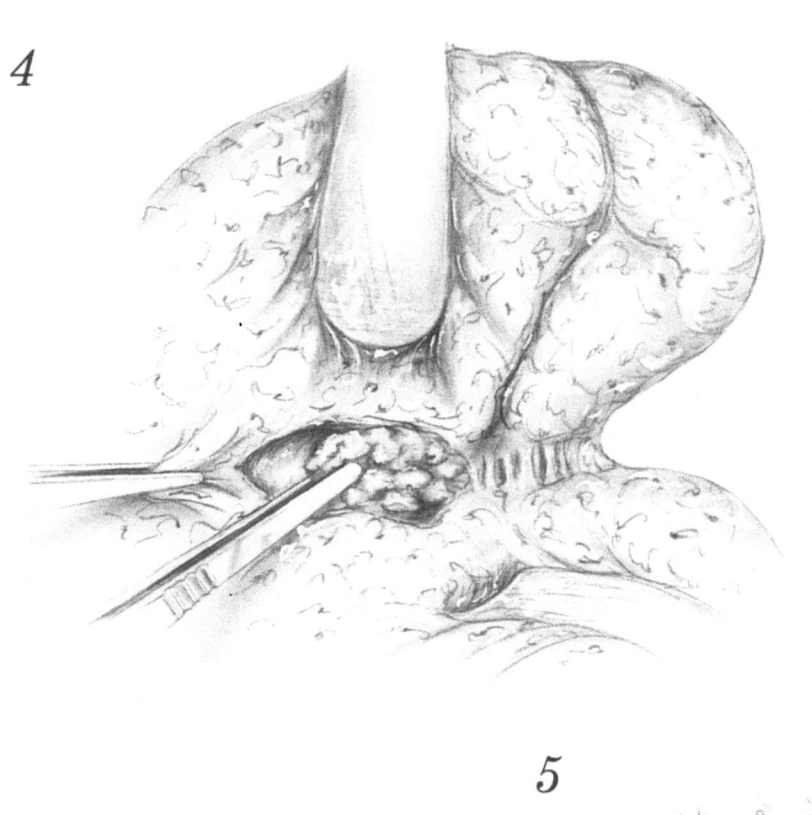

4 The fissure between the right lower lobe and the upper and middle lobes is developed, dissecting the lymph nodes to expose the pulmonary artery in the fissure.

5

5 The branches of the pulmonary artery to the lower lobe are exposed and identified.

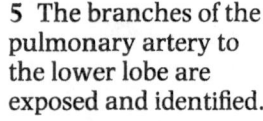
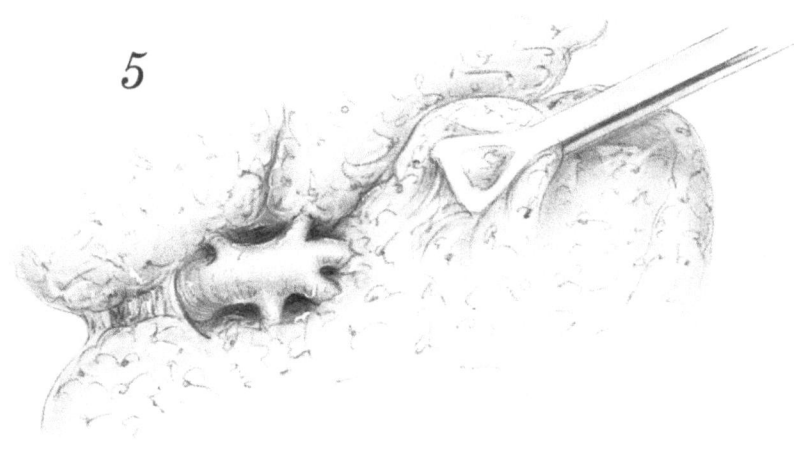

6

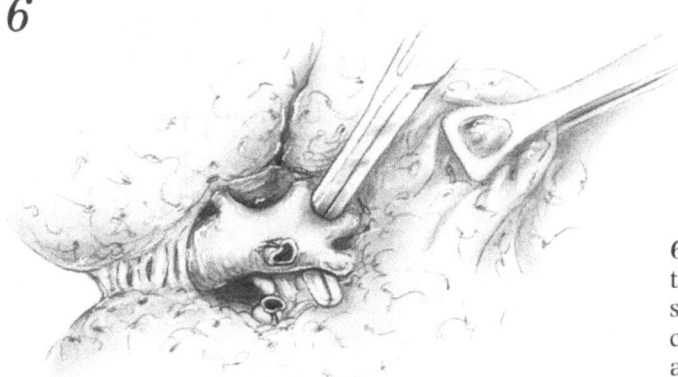

6 The branches are tied and divided, taking the branch to the apical lower segment separately. The branches to the basal segments can be taken together, sparing the middle lobe artery anteriorly.

7

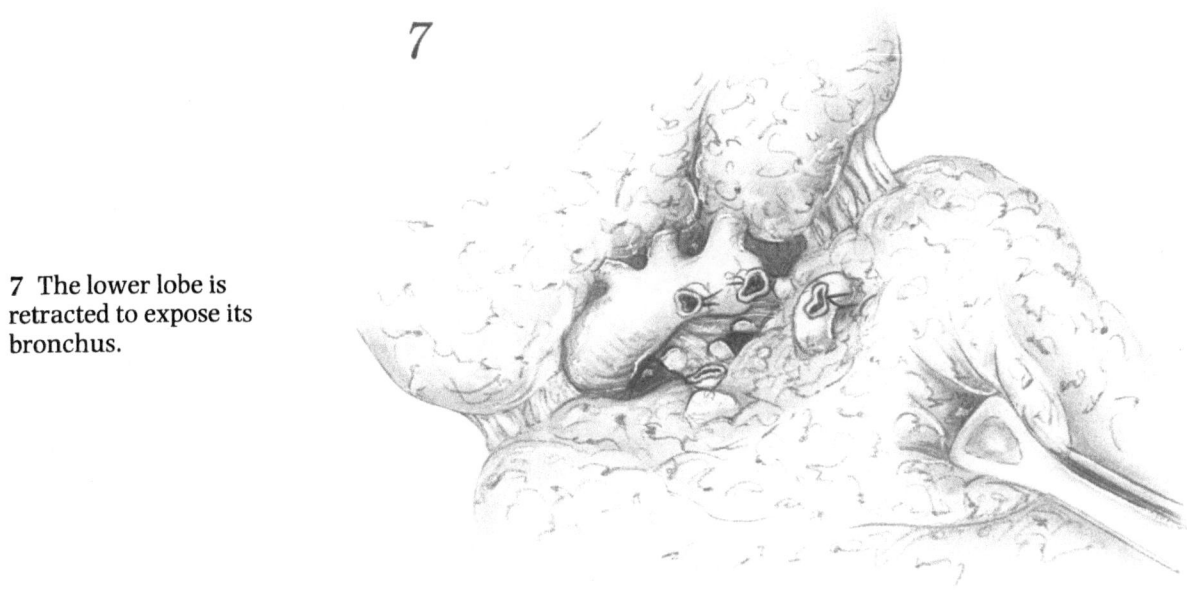

7 The lower lobe is retracted to expose its bronchus.

8

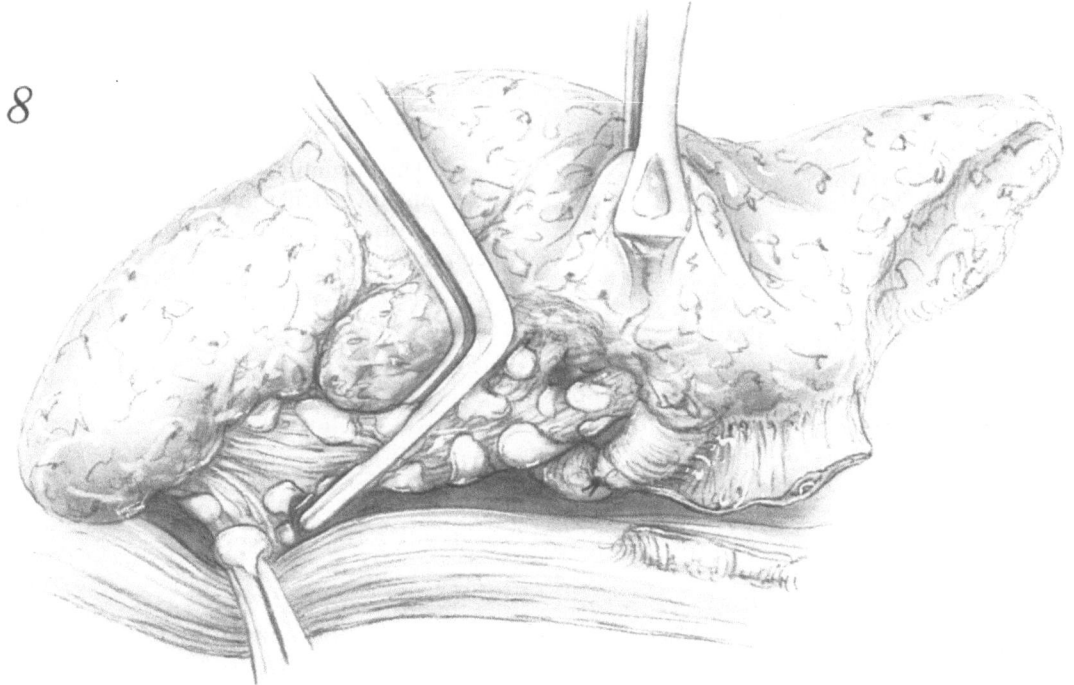

8 The lower lobe bronchus is now clamped obliquely at its origin, flush with the middle lobe bronchus but extending up to the upper lobe bronchus. The oesophagus has been gently retracted.

9

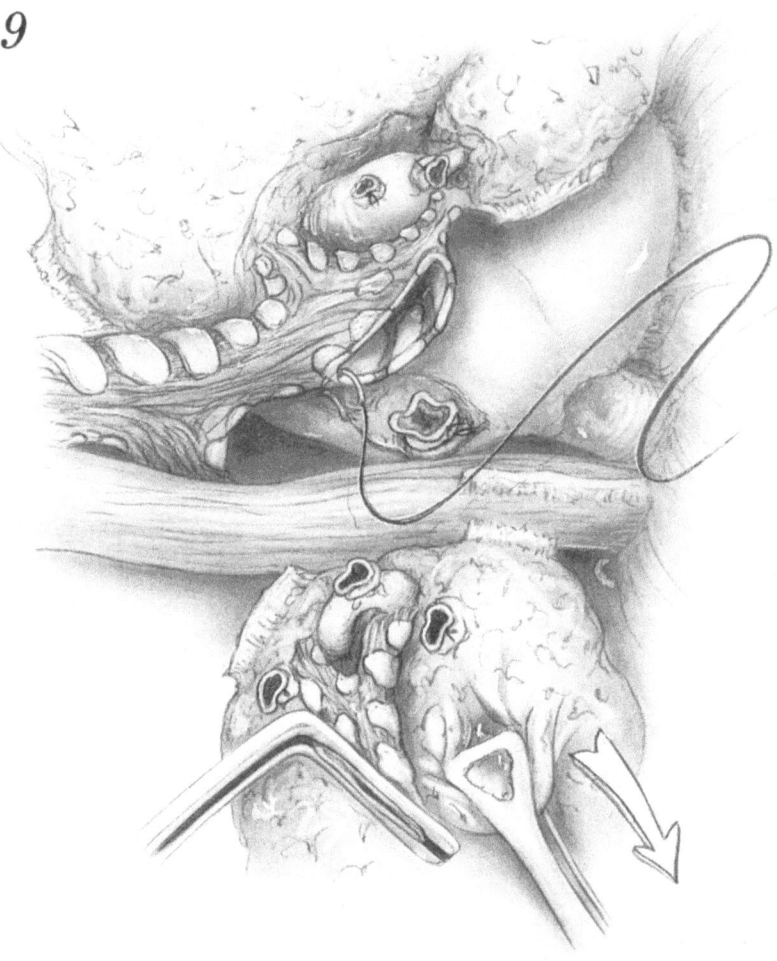

9, 10 The bronchial stump is closed with interrupted vertical mattress sutures covered by a continuous stitch, and the lower lobe has been removed.

10

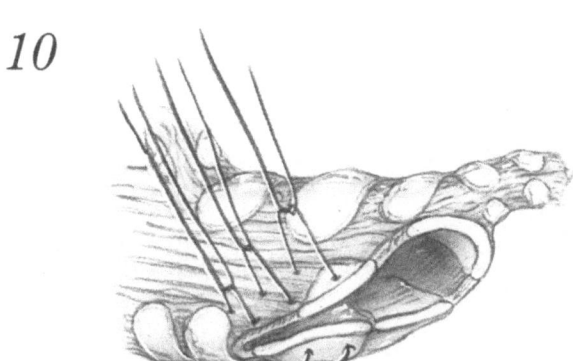

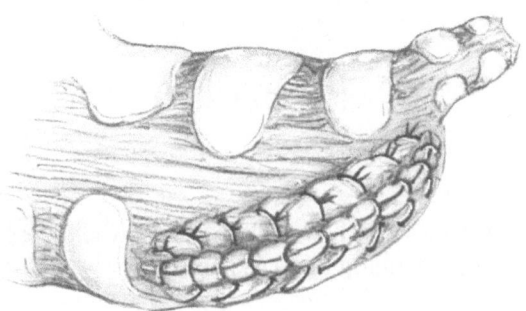

11

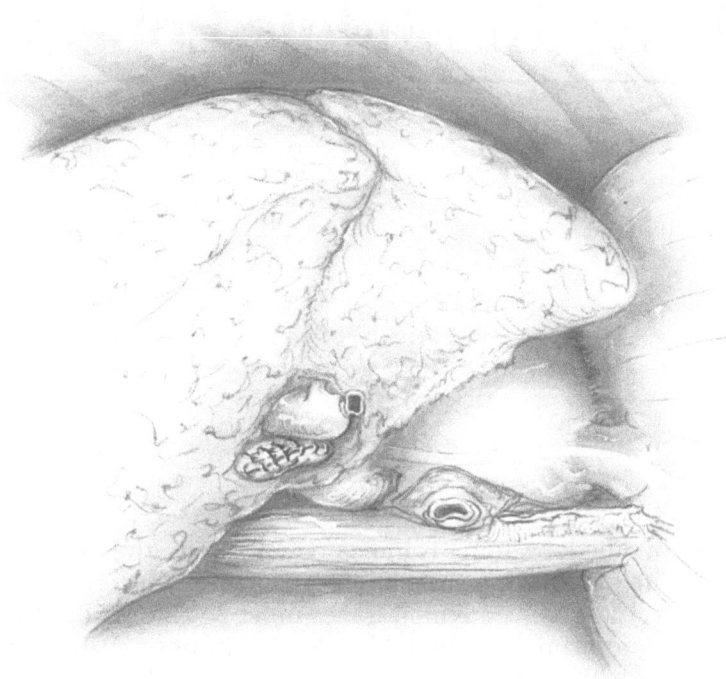

11 The upper and middle lobes are inflated to fill the chest and the chest is closed routinely.

The incision is closed in layers with anterior and posterior drainage tubes, with sideholes, extending up to the apex. The chest drains should not be clamped during transport of the patient back to the ward, and care must be taken that the drains are not dislodged or kinked during movement. Once the patient is back in the ward the chest drains are connected to suction which must have careful control and be capable of high volume suction. Suction should be sufficient to maintain a negative pressure resulting in continuous bubbling throughout the respiratory cycle. Tubes are removed sequentially when all drainage and air leak has stopped.

Prophylactic antibiotics should be discontinued after 24 h. Antibiotics are thereafter only indicated for specific infective problems.

Adequate pain relief should be ensured to permit early and full movement of the shoulder and to allow the patient to co-operate with the physiotherapist in expectoration. Sputum problems are common following pulmonary resection, and if not dealt with promptly, will lead to life-threatening complications such as pulmonary infection. If sputum retention occurs despite adequate analgesia and intensive physiotherapy, suction bronchoscopy may be necessary. The insertion of a minitracheostomy tube through the cricothyroid membrane has largely replaced the performance of formal tracheostomy.

Cardiac dysrhythmias, particularly atrial tachycardias, are common following pulmonary resection, and prophylactic digoxin is often used in the elderly.

With the emphasis on early mobilisation, deep venous thrombosis and pulmonary embolism are now rarities and there is no evidence that low dose heparin is of any value.

7 Right Middle Lobectomy

Right middle lobectomy is indicated whenever the disease process is limited to the right middle lobe. The commonest such indication in the western world is carcinoma of the bronchus. The tumour and involved lymph nodes must be confined to the lobe, and lines of resection through vessels and bronchus should be clear of tumour. When undertaken for pulmonary sepsis, pre-operative physiotherapy may produce a temporary but important improvement in the patient's condition and help minimise post-operative sputum difficulties. All patients should be instructed pre-operatively in the physiotherapy manoeuvres which will be undertaken post-operatively. Prophylactic antibiotics commenced with the premedication and continued for 24 h have been shown to reduce the incidence of wound infection but will have no influence on the more serious problems of chest infection and infection of the pleural space.

An endobronchial tube passed by the anaesthetist will allow single lung ventilation. The collapse of the lung on the side of surgery will minimise the competing aims of surgeon and anaesthetist.

1

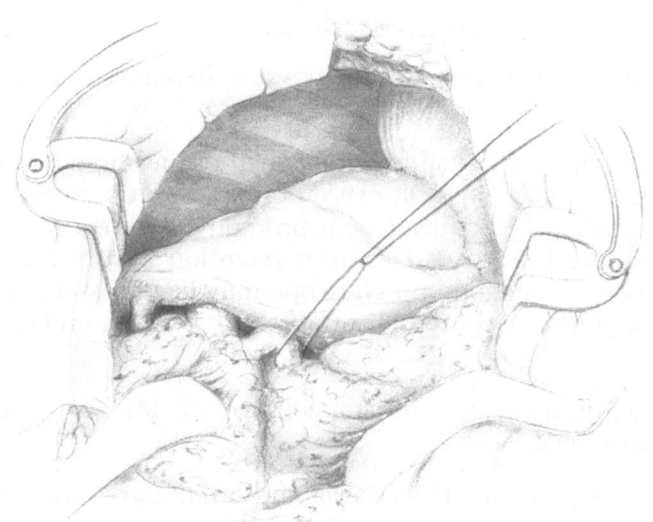

1 The right chest has been entered by stripping the lower border of the fifth rib, and the middle lobe tributary of the right superior pulmonary vein is dissected and ligated.

2

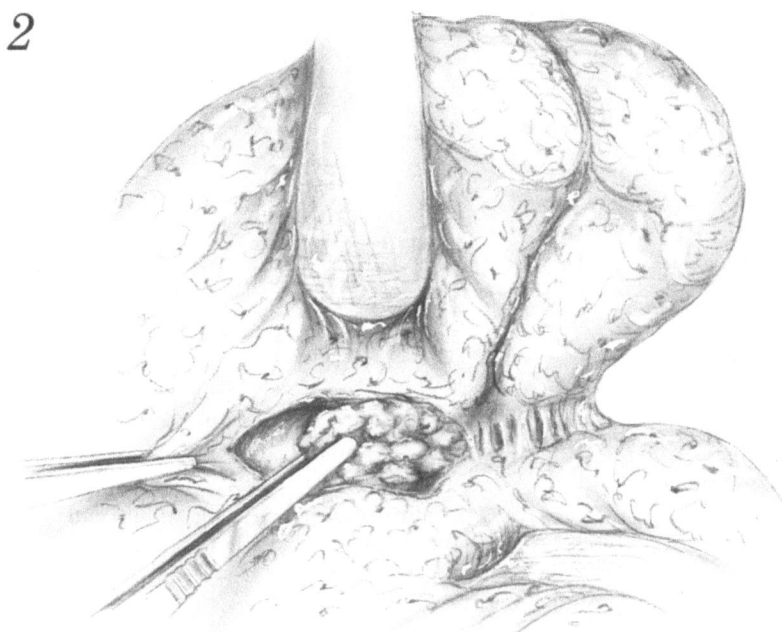

2 The fissure between the right lower lobe and the upper and middle lobes is developed, dissecting the lymph nodes to expose the pulmonary artery in the fissure.

3

3 When the pulmonary artery has been fully dissected out in the fissure, the right middle lobe artery is ligated and divided.

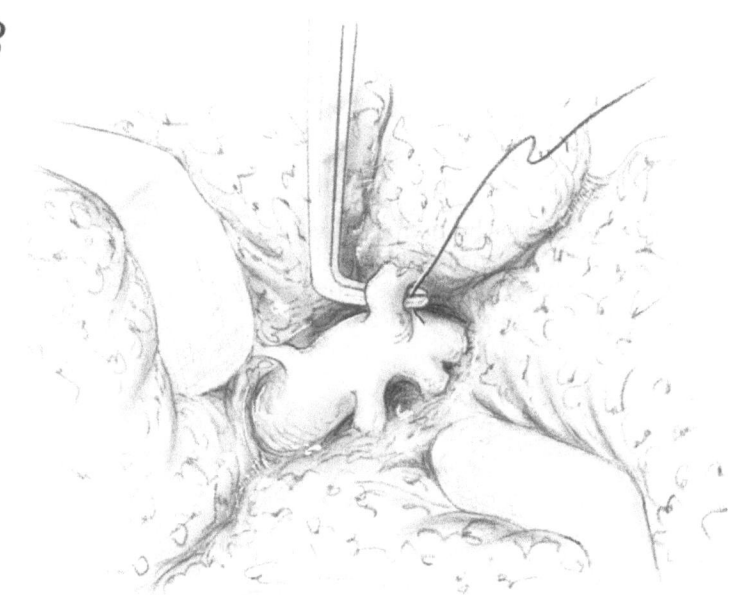

4

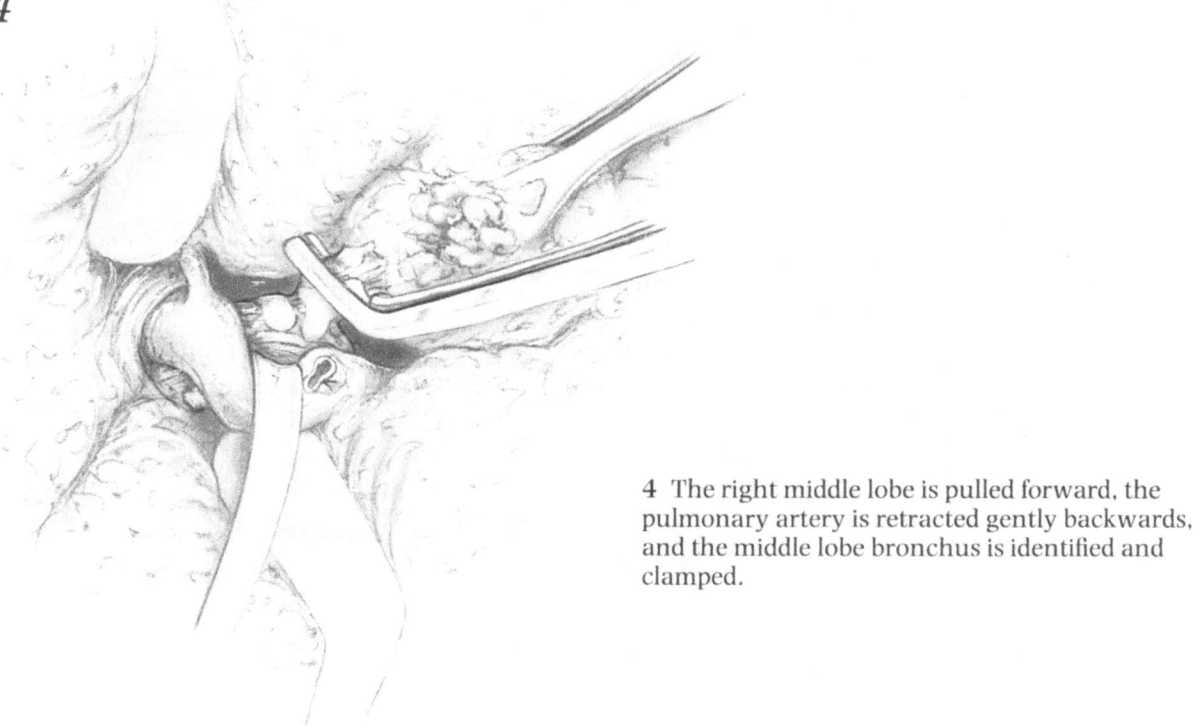

4 The right middle lobe is pulled forward, the pulmonary artery is retracted gently backwards, and the middle lobe bronchus is identified and clamped.

5

5 The middle lobe bronchus is divided and closed in routine fashion by interrupted vertical mattress sutures covered by a continuous stitch.

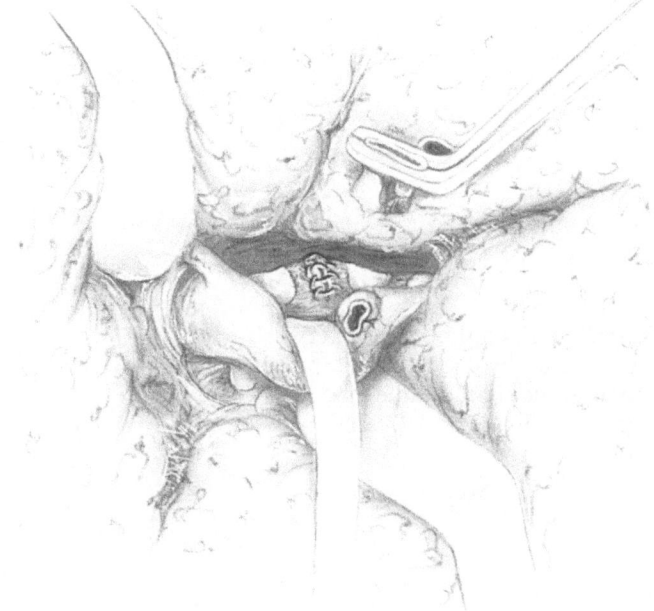

6

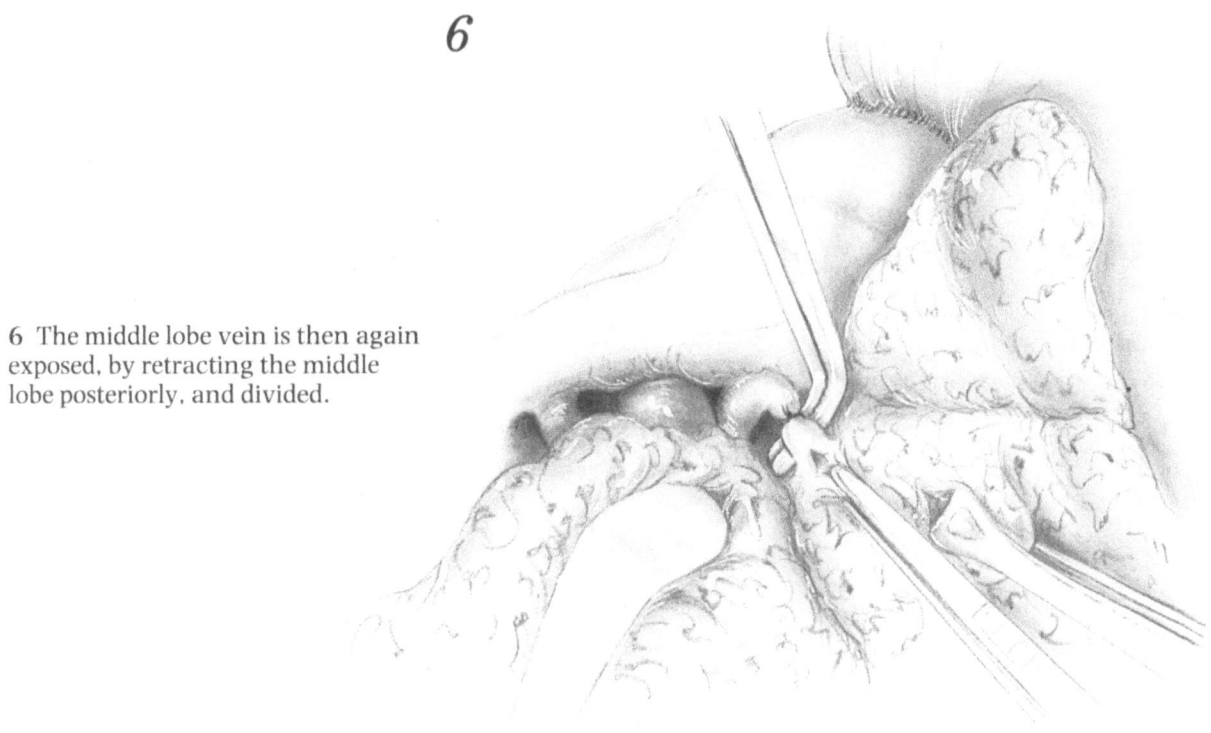

6 The middle lobe vein is then again exposed, by retracting the middle lobe posteriorly, and divided.

7

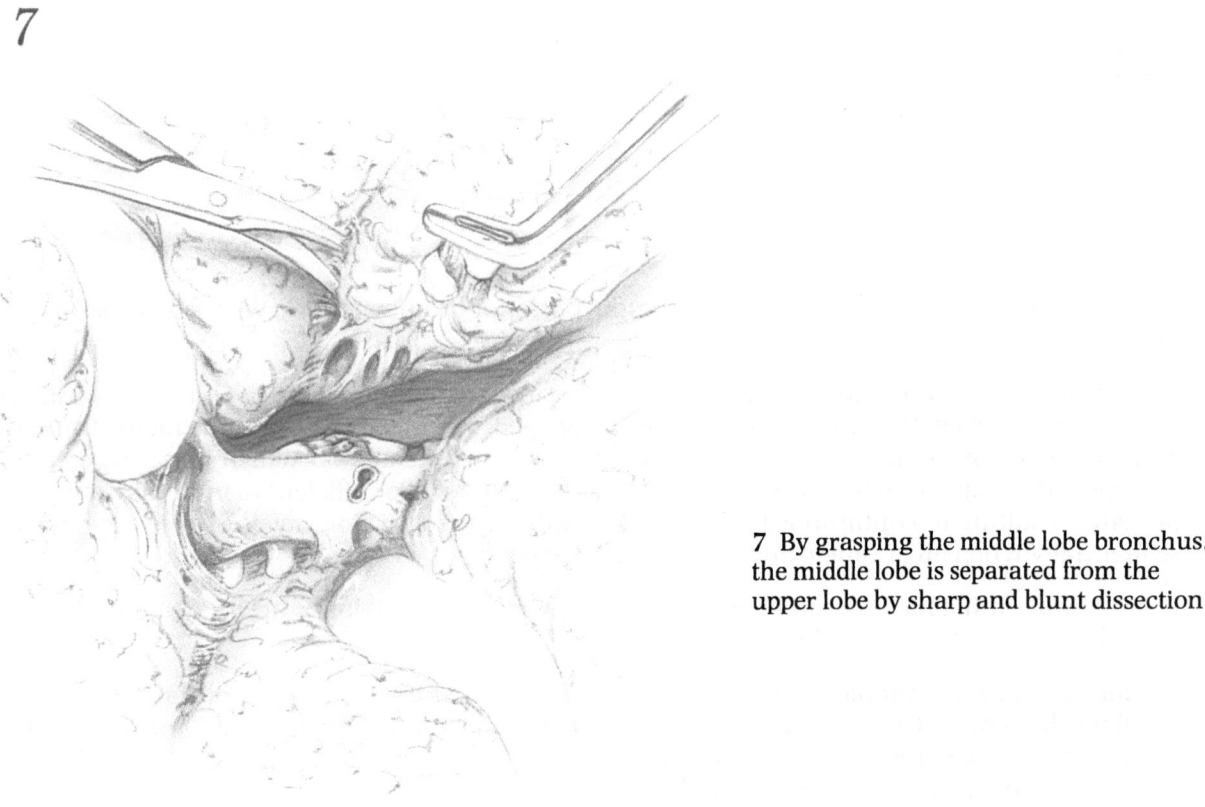

7 By grasping the middle lobe bronchus, the middle lobe is separated from the upper lobe by sharp and blunt dissection.

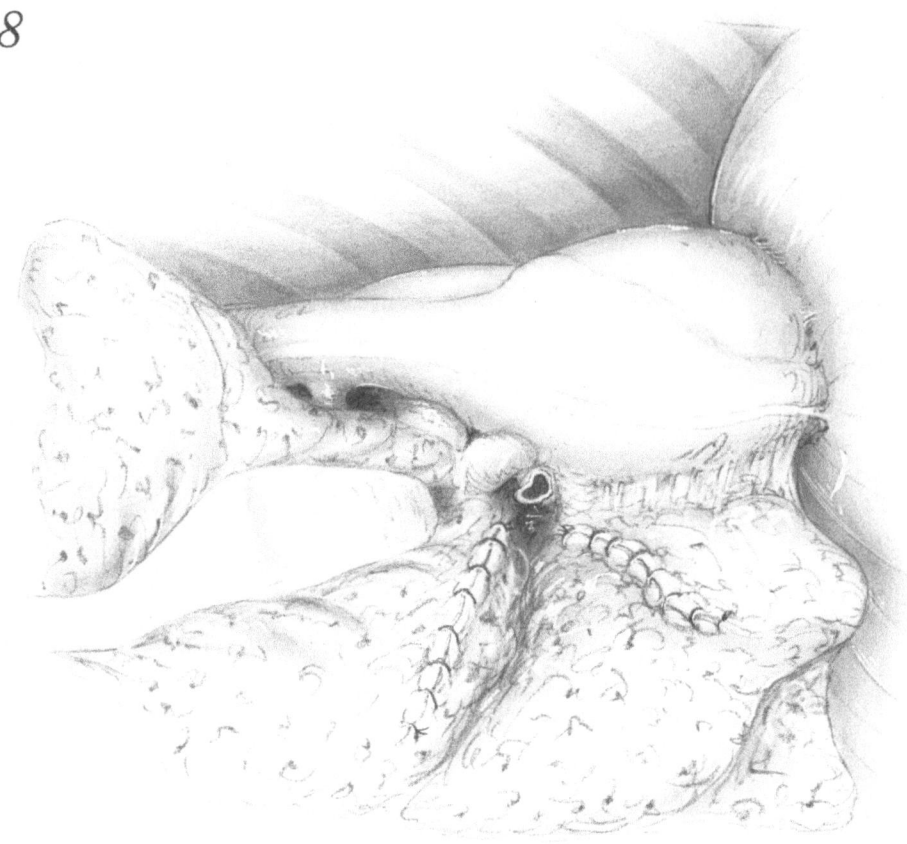

8 The resulting raw surfaces on the upper and lower lobes are then sutured in two layers with an absorbable suture. The chest is then closed routinely.

The incision is closed in layers with anterior and posterior drainage tubes, with sideholes, extending up to the apex.

The chest drains should not be clamped during transport of the patient back to the ward, and care must be taken that the drains are not dislodged or kinked during movement. Once the patient is back in the ward the chest drains are connected to suction which must have careful control and be capable of high volume suction. Suction should be sufficient to maintain a negative pressure resulting in continuous bubbling throughout the respiratory cycle. Tubes are removed sequentially when all drainage and air leak has stopped.

Prophylactic antibiotics should be discontinued after 24 h. Antibiotics are thereafter only indicated for specific infective problems.

Adequate pain relief should be ensured to permit early and full movement of the shoulder and to allow the patient to co-operate with the physiotherapist in expectoration. Sputum problems are common following pulmonary resection, and if not dealt with promptly, will lead to life-threatening complications such as pulmonary infection. If sputum retention occurs despite adequate analgesia and intensive physiotherapy, suction bronchoscopy may be necessary. The insertion of a minitracheostomy tube through the cricothyroid membrane has largely replaced the performance of formal tracheostomy.

Cardiac dysrhythmias, particularly atrial tachycardias, are common following pulmonary resection, and prophylactic digoxin is often used in the elderly.

With the emphasis on early mobilisation, deep venous thrombosis and pulmonary embolism are now rarities and there is no evidence that low dose heparin is of any value.

8 Right Middle and Lower Lobectomy

Right middle and lower lobectomy is indicated whenever the disease process is limited to the right middle and lower lobes. The commonest such indication in the western world is carcinoma of the bronchus. The tumour and involved lymph nodes must be confined to the lobes, and lines of resection through vessels and bronchus should be clear of tumour. When undertaken for pulmonary sepsis, pre-operative physiotherapy may produce a temporary but important improvement in the patient's condition and help minimise post-operative sputum difficulties. All patients should be instructed pre-operatively in the physiotherapy manoeuvres which will be undertaken post-operatively. Prophylactic antibiotics commenced with the premedication and continued for 24 h have been shown to reduce the incidence of wound infection but will have no influence on the more serious problems of chest infection and infection of the pleural space.

An endobronchial tube passed by the anaesthetist will allow single lung ventilation. The collapse of the lung on the side of surgery will minimise the competing aims of surgeon and anaesthetist.

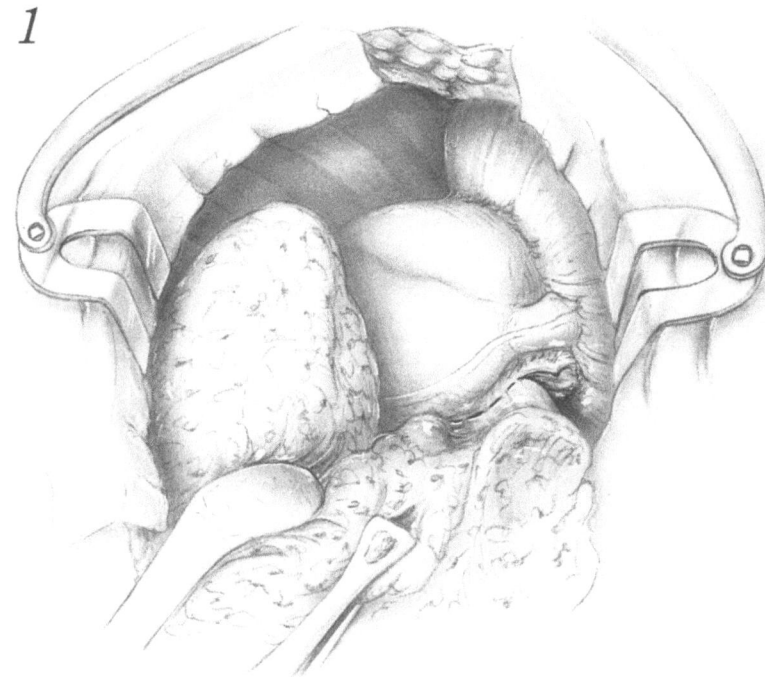

1

1 The chest has been opened by stripping the lower border of the fifth or sixth rib. The pulmonary ligament is divided upwards to the inferior pulmonary vein.

2 The inferior pulmonary vein is secured at the pericardial reflection. (*Inset*: the middle lobe tributary of the superior pulmonary vein is also secured.)

2

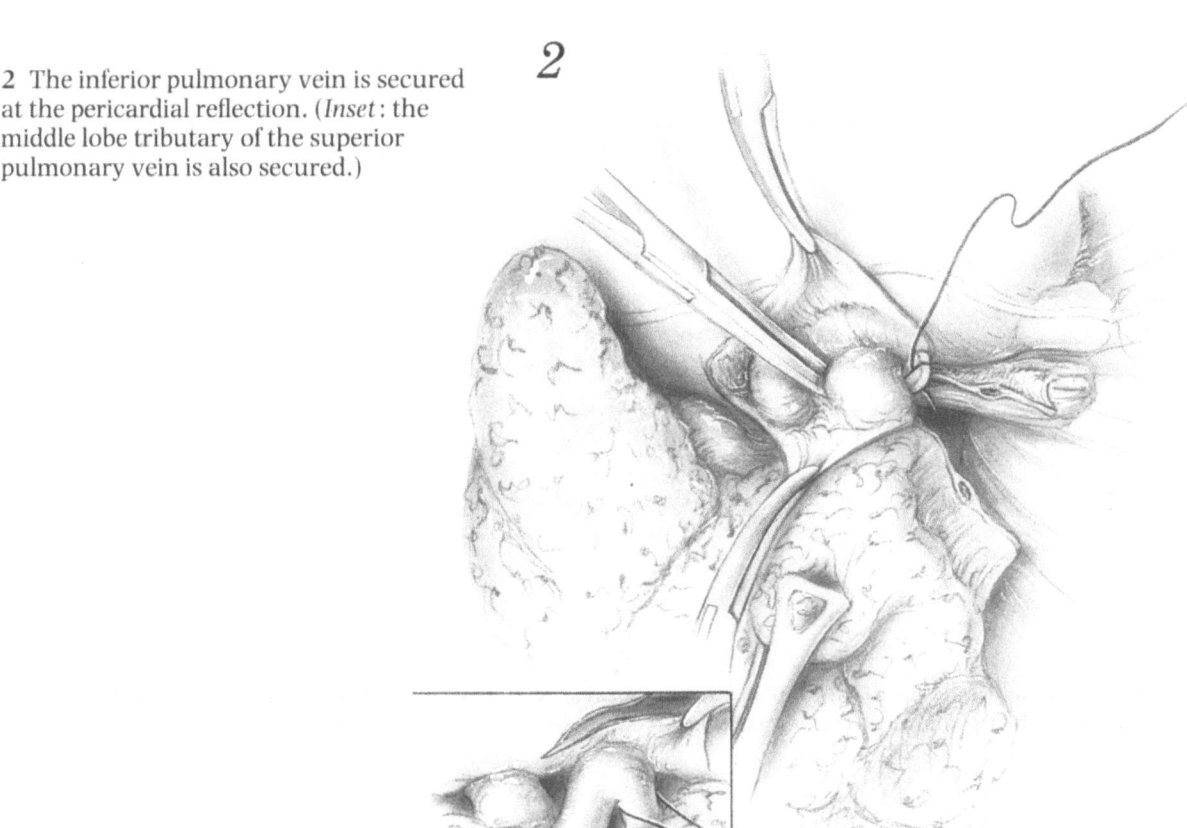

3

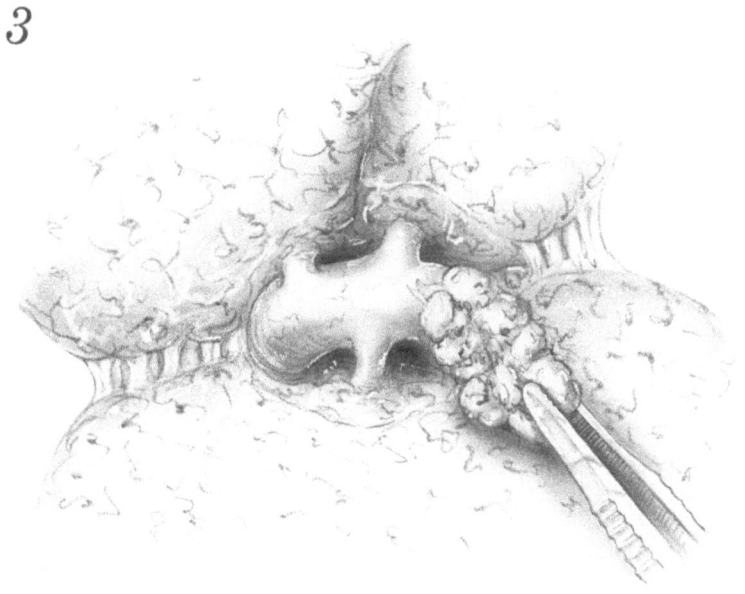

3 The fissure is developed by dissecting the lymph nodes overlying the pulmonary artery downwards and exposing the branches of the pulmonary artery to the middle and lower lobes.

4

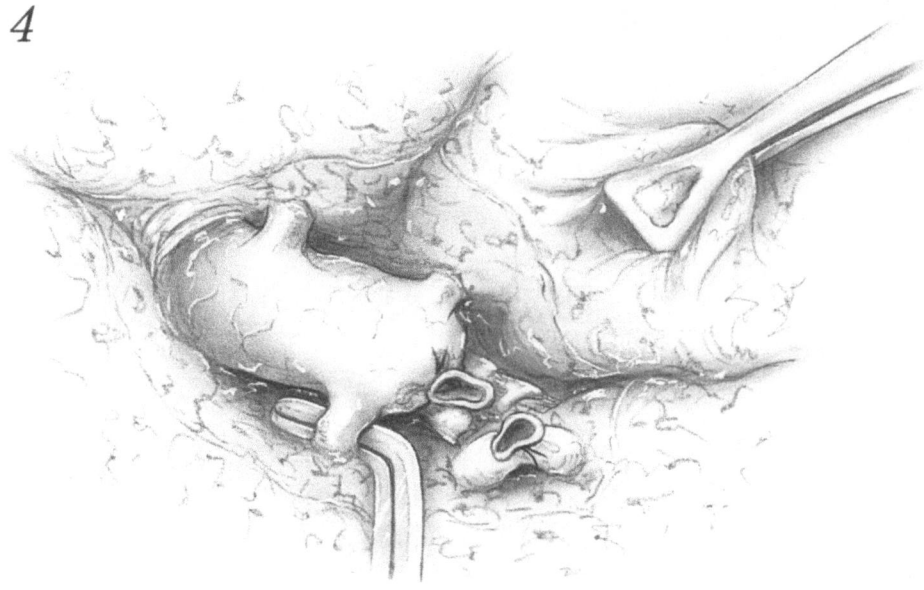

4 The branches of the pulmonary artery to the basal segments of the lower lobe have been tied and divided, and the apical lower branch is being tied and divided.

5

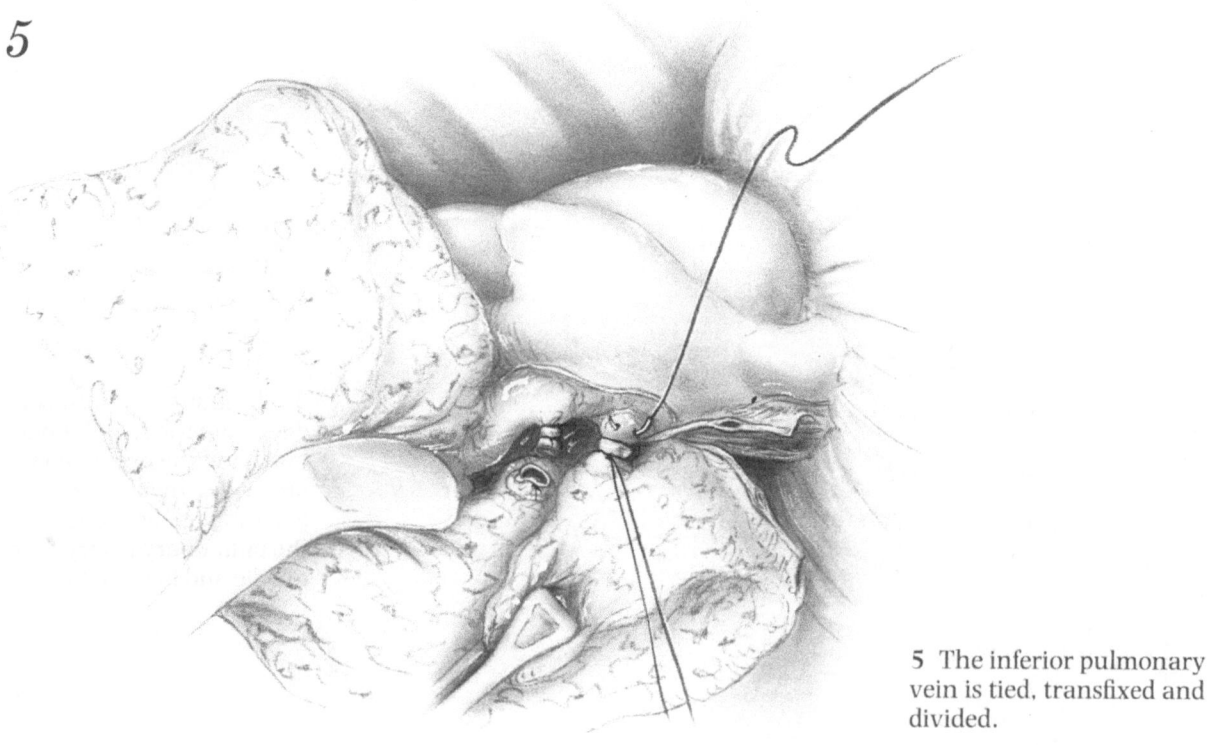

5 The inferior pulmonary vein is tied, transfixed and divided.

6

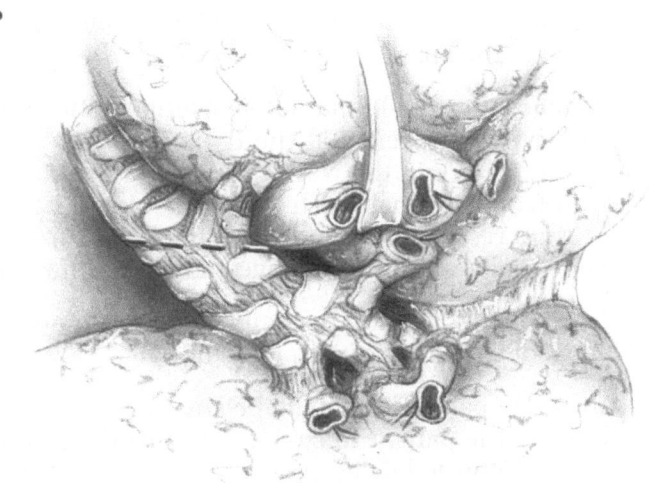

6 The pulmonary artery is retracted forwards and the bronchus to the middle and lower lobes is divided immediately below its upper lobe division, the line of division being oblique.

7

7 The middle and lower lobes have been removed and the bronchial stump is closed routinely with interrupted mattress sutures covered by an over-and-over stitch. The chest is then closed routinely.

The incision is closed in layers with anterior and posterior drainage tubes, with sideholes, extending up to the apex.

The chest drains should not be clamped during transport of the patient back to the ward, and care must be taken that the drains are not dislodged or kinked during movement. Once the patient is back in the ward the chest drains are connected to suction which must have careful control and be capable of high volume suction. Suction should be sufficient to maintain a negative pressure resulting in continuous bubbling throughout the respiratory cycle. Tubes are removed sequentially when all drainage and air leak has stopped.

Prophylactic antibiotics should be discontinued after 24 h. Antibiotics are thereafter only indicated for specific infective problems.

Adequate pain relief should be ensured to permit early and full movement of the shoulder and to allow the patient to co-operate with the physiotherapist in expectoration. Sputum problems are common following pulmonary resection, and if not dealt with promptly, will lead to life-threatening complications such as pulmonary infection. If sputum retention occurs despite adequate analgesia and intensive physiotherapy, suction bronchoscopy may be necessary. The insertion of a minitracheostomy tube through the cricothyroid membrane has largely replaced the performance of formal tracheostomy.

Cardiac dysrhythmias, particularly atrial tachycardias, are common following pulmonary resection, and prophylactic digoxin is often used in the elderly.

With the emphasis on early mobilisation, deep venous thrombosis and pulmonary embolism are now rarities and there is no evidence that low dose heparin is of any value.

9 Left Lower Lobectomy

Left lower lobectomy is indicated whenever the disease process is limited to the left lower lobe. The commonest such indication in the western world is carcinoma of the bronchus. The tumour and involved lymph nodes must be confined to the lobe, and lines of resection through vessels and bronchus should be clear of tumour. When undertaken for pulmonary sepsis, pre-operative physiotherapy may produce a temporary but important improvement in the patient's condition and help minimise post-operative sputum difficulties. All patients should be instructed pre-operatively in the physiotherapy manoeuvres which will be undertaken post-operatively. Prophylactic antibiotics commenced with the premedication and continued for 24 h have been shown to reduce the incidence of wound infection but will have no influence on the more serious problems of chest infection and infection of the pleural space.

An endobronchial tube passed by the anaesthetist will allow single lung ventilation. The collapse of the lung on the side of surgery will minimise the competing aims of surgeon and anaesthetist.

1

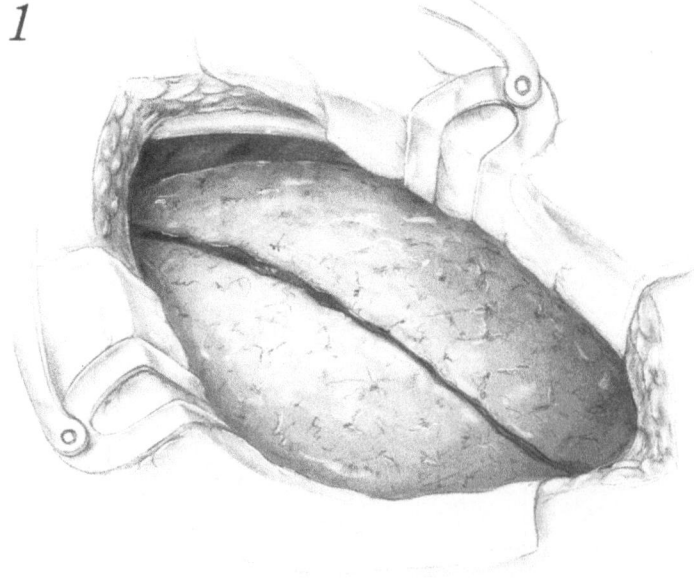

1 The chest has been opened by stripping the periosteum off the lower border of the fifth rib (see Left Upper Lobectomy).

2

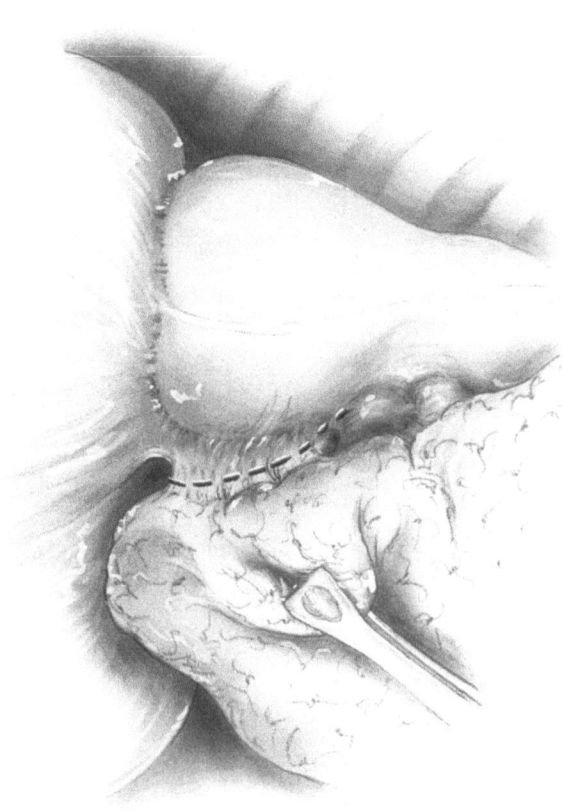

2 The pulmonary ligament is incised from the diaphragm to the inferior pulmonary vein.

3

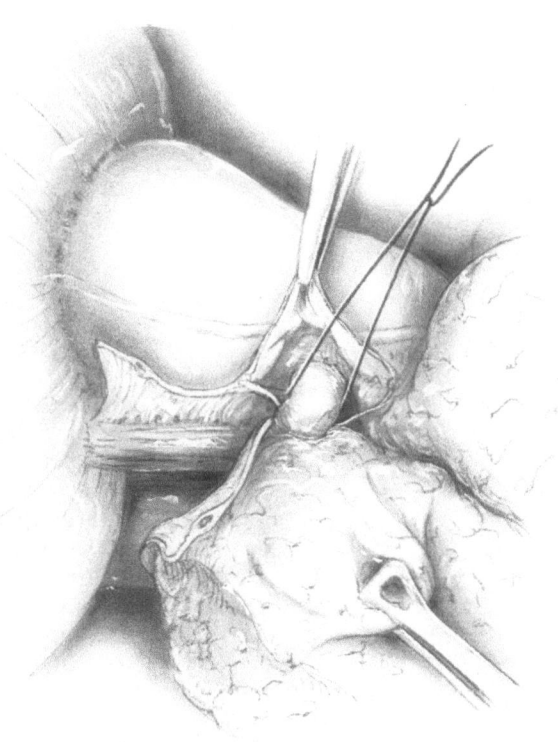

3 The pericardium surrounding the inferior pulmonary vein is opened and the inferior pulmonary vein is tied as a first step.

4

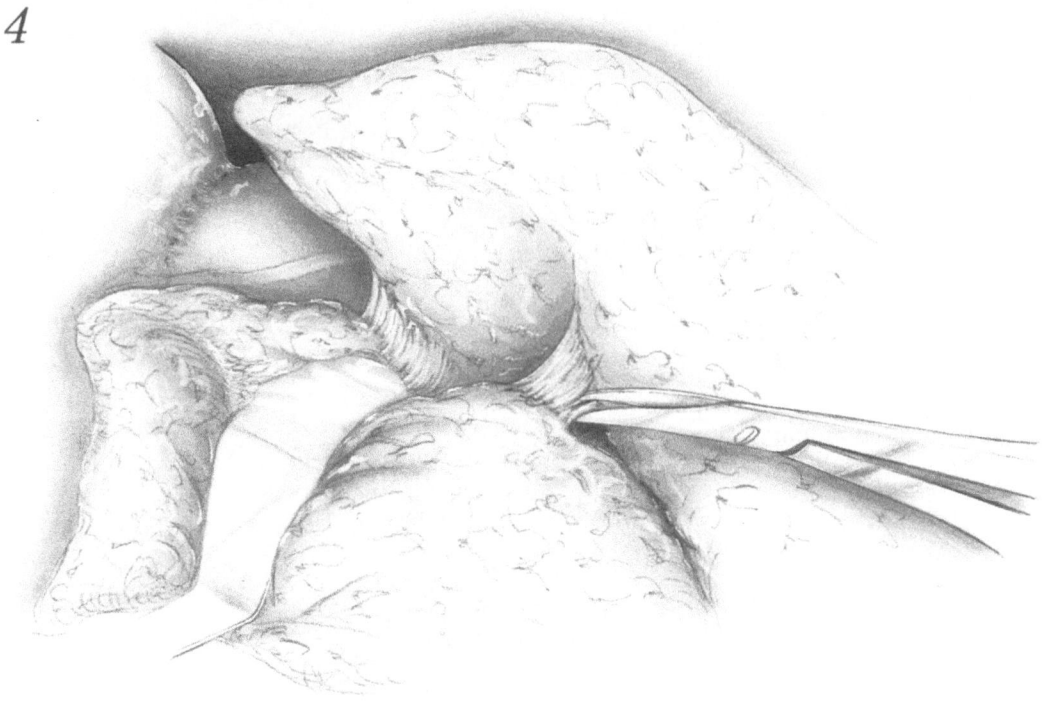

4 The fissure is developed by sharp dissection.

5

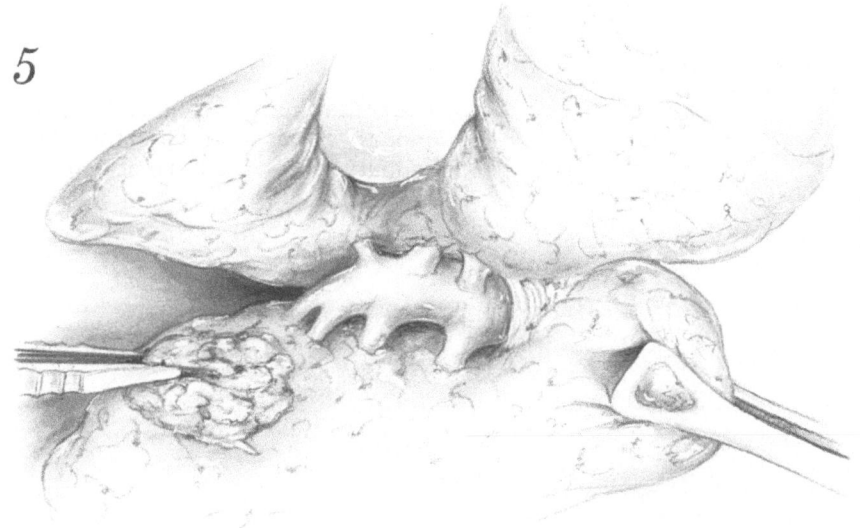

5 The branches of the pulmonary artery to the lower lobe are exposed by dissecting the glands in the fissure downwards with the lower lobe.

6

6 The branches to the basal segments of the lower lobe may be taken together or separately, but the branch to the apical segment of the lower lobe has to be taken separately so as not to compromise the lingular branches to the upper lobe.

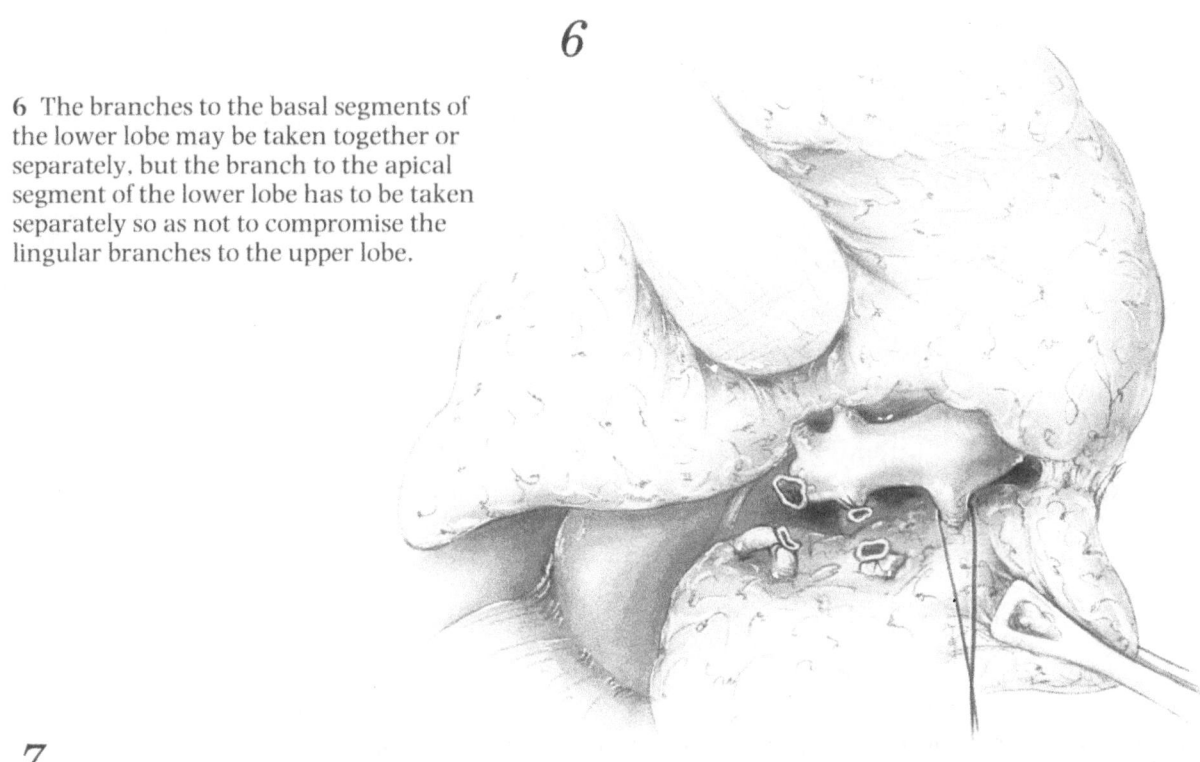

7

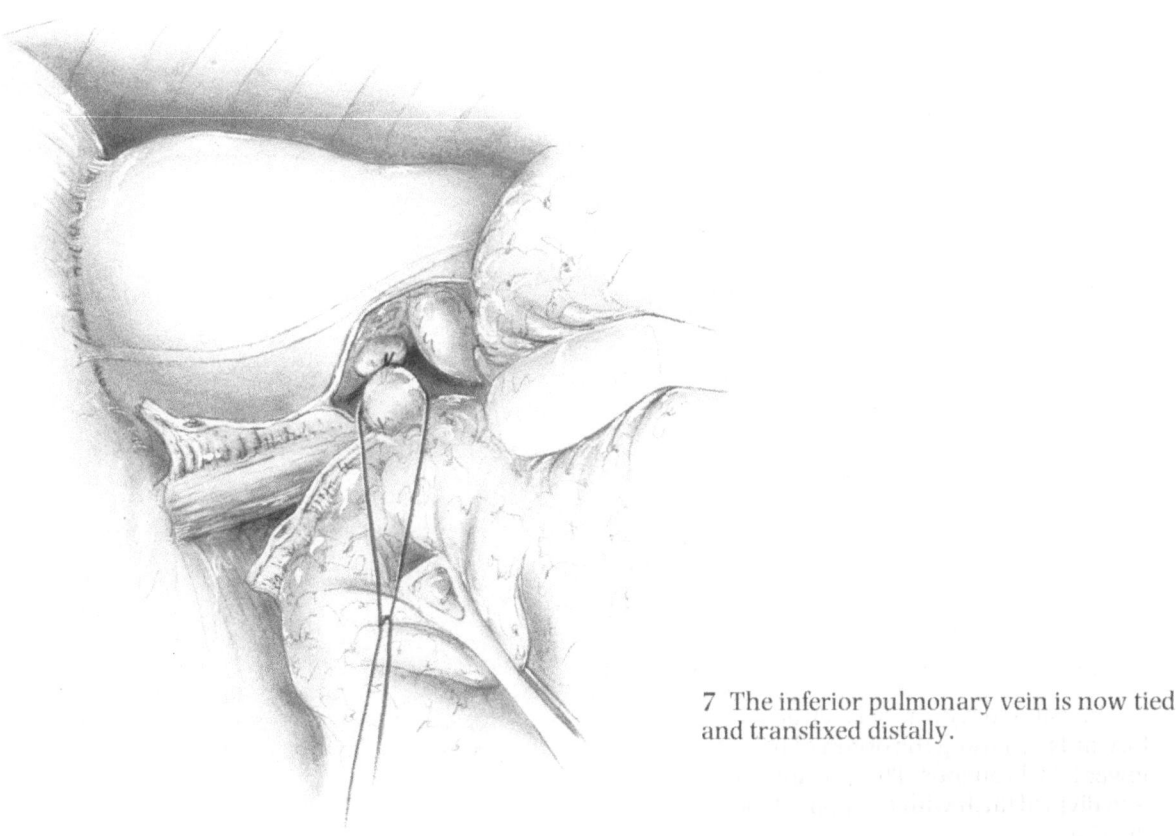

7 The inferior pulmonary vein is now tied and transfixed distally.

8

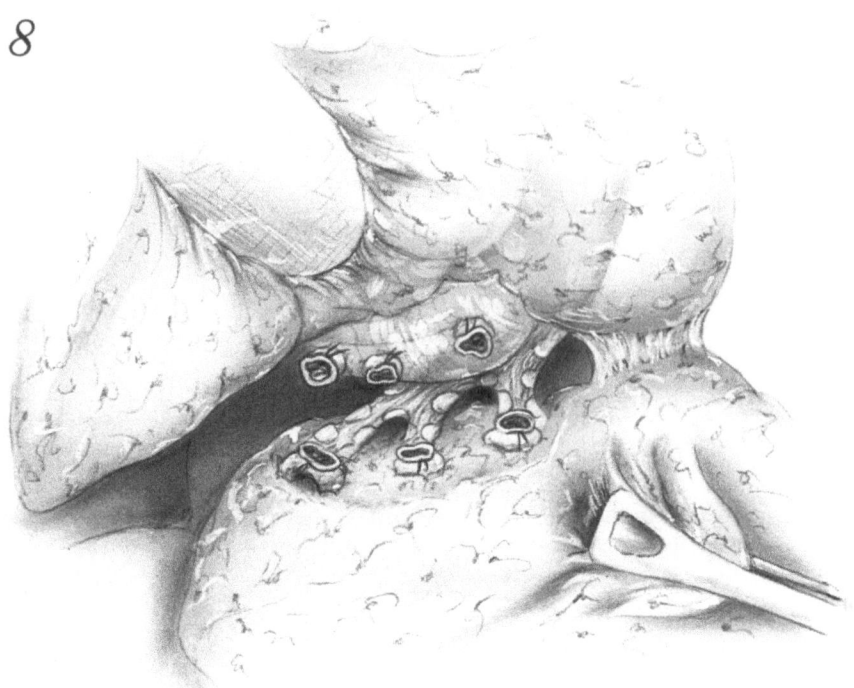

8 The lower lobe is now finally separated from the upper lobe, and behind the pulmonary artery the lower lobe bronchus is exposed.

9

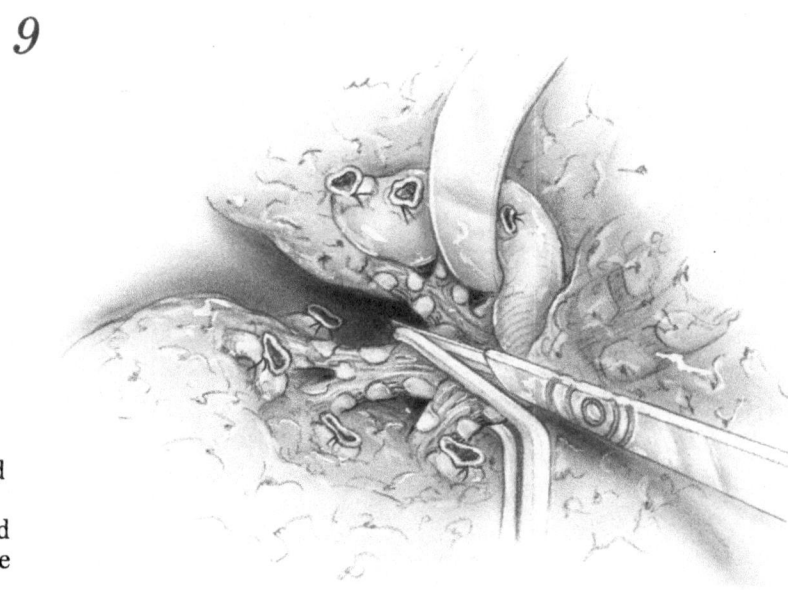

9 The pulmonary artery is retracted forwards, exposing the origin of the lower lobe bronchus. This is clamped and divided flush with the upper lobe division.

10 The lower lobe has been removed and the origin of the lower lobe bronchus is clearly seen.

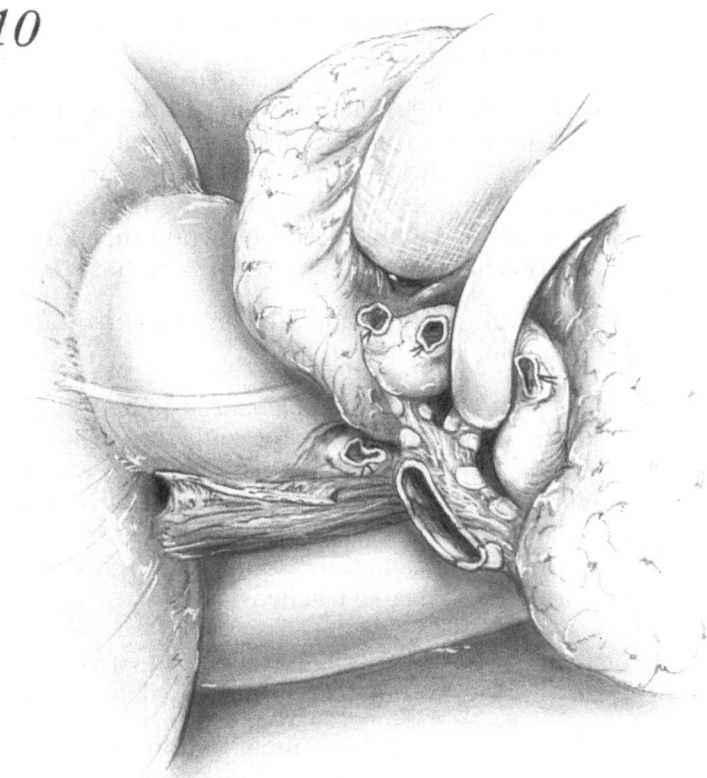

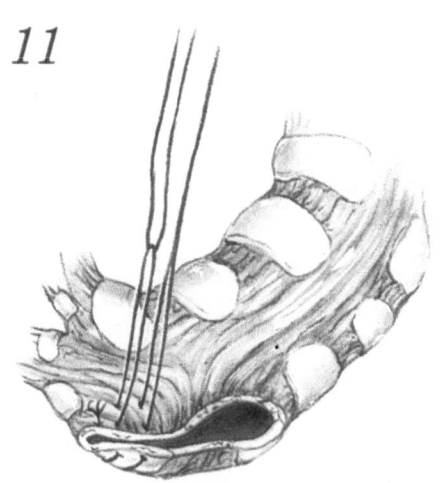

11 The origin of the lower lobe bronchus is closed with interrupted vertical mattress sutures covered by an over-and-over stitch.

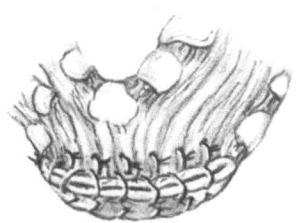

The incision is closed in layers with anterior and posterior drainage tubes, with sideholes, extending up to the apex.

The chest drains should not be clamped during transport of the patient back to the ward, and care must be taken that the drains are not dislodged or kinked during movement. Once the patient is back in the ward the chest drains are connected to suction which must have careful control and be capable of high volume suction. Suction should be sufficient to maintain a negative pressure resulting in continuous bubbling throughout the respiratory cycle. Tubes are removed sequentially when all drainage and air leak has stopped.

Prophylactic antibiotics should be discontinued after 24 h. Antibiotics are thereafter only indicated for specific infective problems.

Adequate pain relief should be ensured to permit early and full movement of the shoulder and to allow the patient to co-operate with the physiotherapist in expectoration. Sputum problems are common following pulmonary resection, and if not dealt with promptly, will lead to life-threatening complications such as pulmonary infection. If sputum retention occurs despite adequate analgesia and intensive physiotherapy, suction bronchoscopy may be necessary. The insertion of a minitracheostomy tube through the cricothyroid membrane has largely replaced the performance of formal tracheostomy.

Cardiac dysrhythmias, particularly atrial tachycardias, are common following pulmonary resection, and prophylactic digoxin is often used in the elderly.

With the emphasis on early mobilisation, deep venous thrombosis and pulmonary embolism are now rarities and there is no evidence that low dose heparin is of any value.

10 Left Upper Lobectomy

This resection is indicated whenever the disease process is limited to the left upper lobe. The commonest such indication in the western world is carcinoma of the bronchus. The tumour and involved lymph nodes must be confined to the lobe, and lines of resection through vessels and bronchus should be clear of tumour. When undertaken for pulmonary sepsis, pre-operative physiotherapy may produce a temporary but important improvement in the patient's condition and help minimise post-operative sputum difficulties. All patients should be instructed pre-operatively in the physiotherapy manoeuvres which will be undertaken post-operatively. Prophylactic antibiotics commenced with the premedication and continued for 24 h have been shown to reduce the incidence of wound infection but will have no influence on the more serious problems of chest infection and infection of the pleural space.

An endobronchial tube passed by the anaesthetist will allow single lung ventilation. The collapse of the lung on the side of surgery will minimise the competing aims of surgeon and anaesthetist.

1

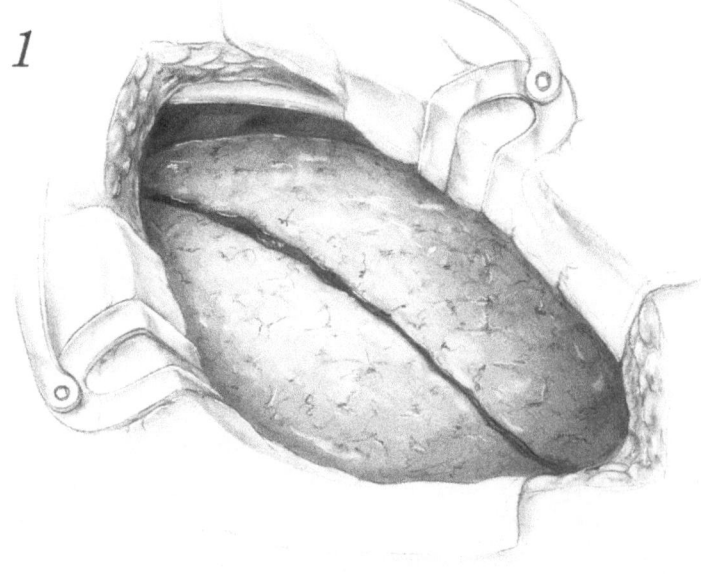

1 The chest has been opened by stripping the periosteum off the lower border of the fifth rib.

2

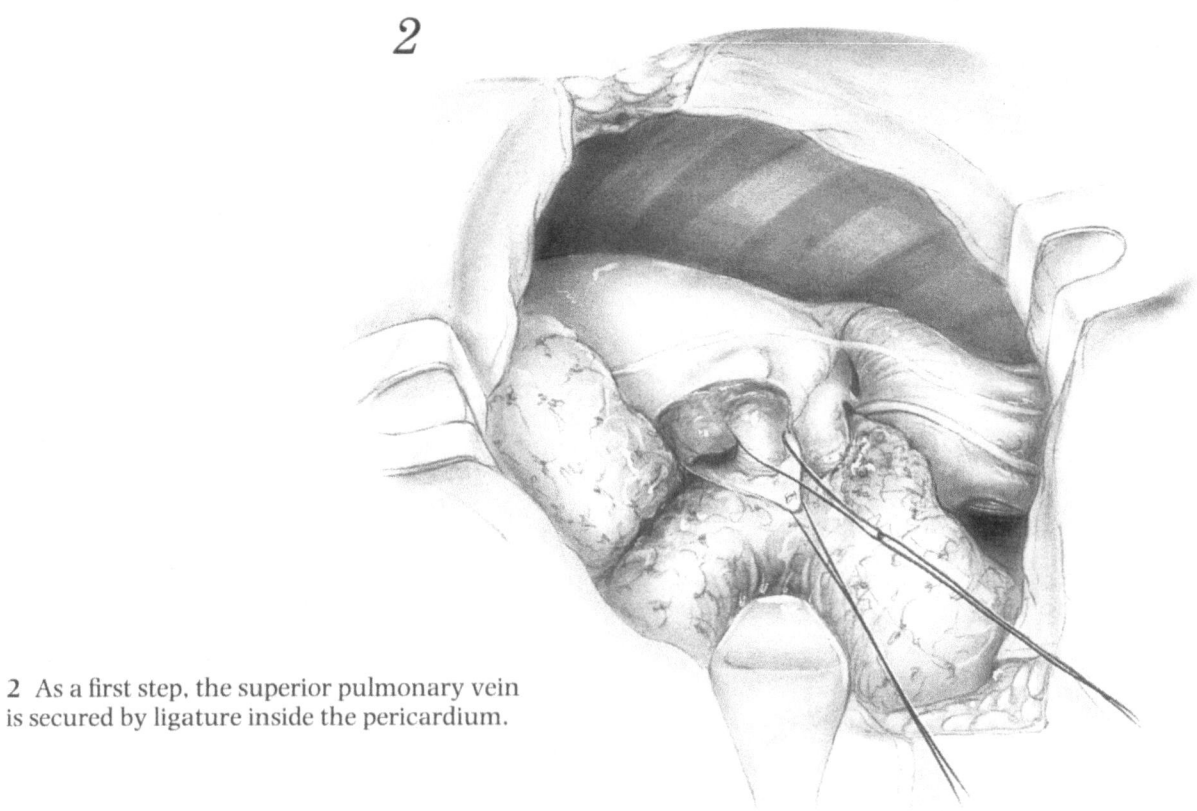

2 As a first step, the superior pulmonary vein is secured by ligature inside the pericardium.

3

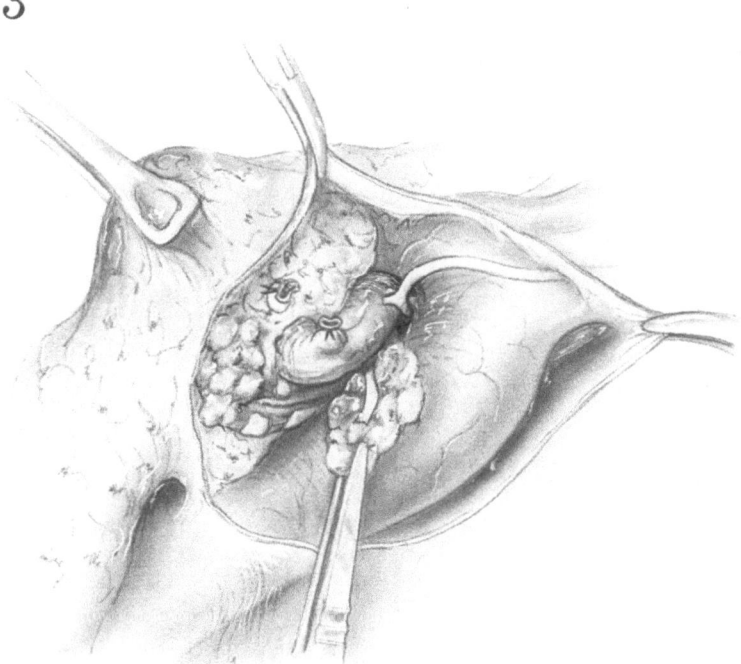

3 The fascia overlying the aorta has been incised, the left vagus nerve has been divided below its recurrent branch and the branches of the pulmonary artery to the upper lobe have been tied and divided, taking the lymph nodes and distal end of the vagus downwards and forwards.

4

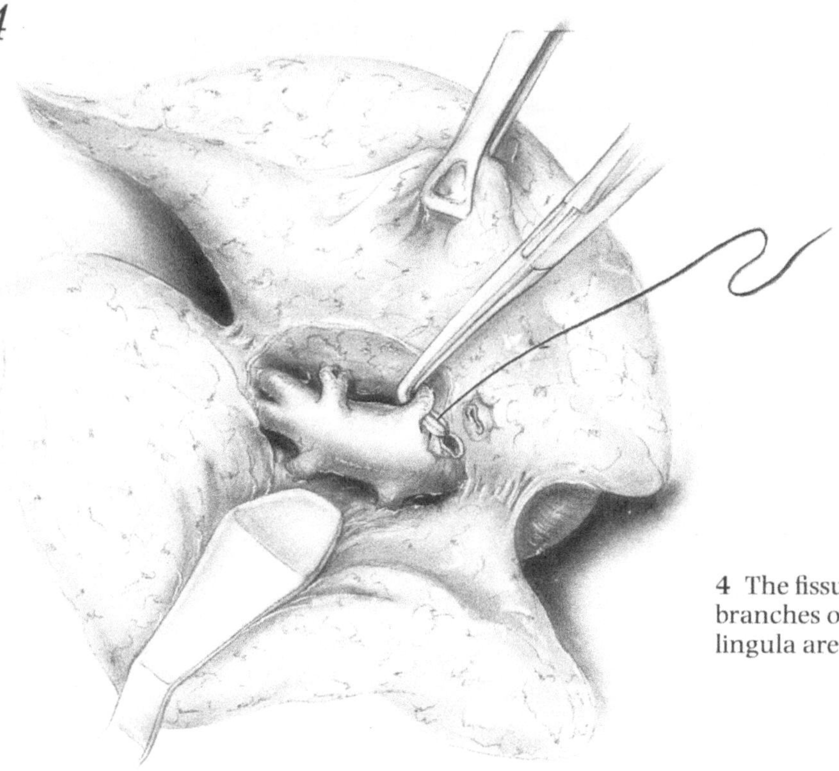

4 The fissure has been developed and the branches of the pulmonary artery to the lingula are identified, under-run and tied.

5

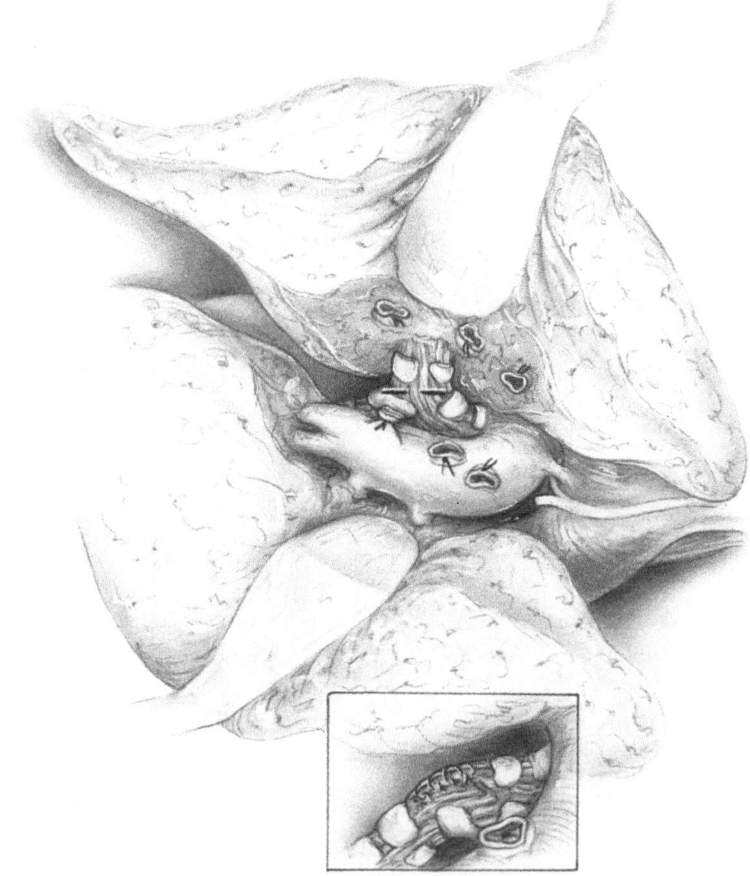

5 After all the branches of the pulmonary artery to the upper lobe have been tied and divided, the descending pulmonary artery is retracted with a dissecting swab, exposing the left upper lobe bronchus at its origin. It is divided and closed (*inset*).

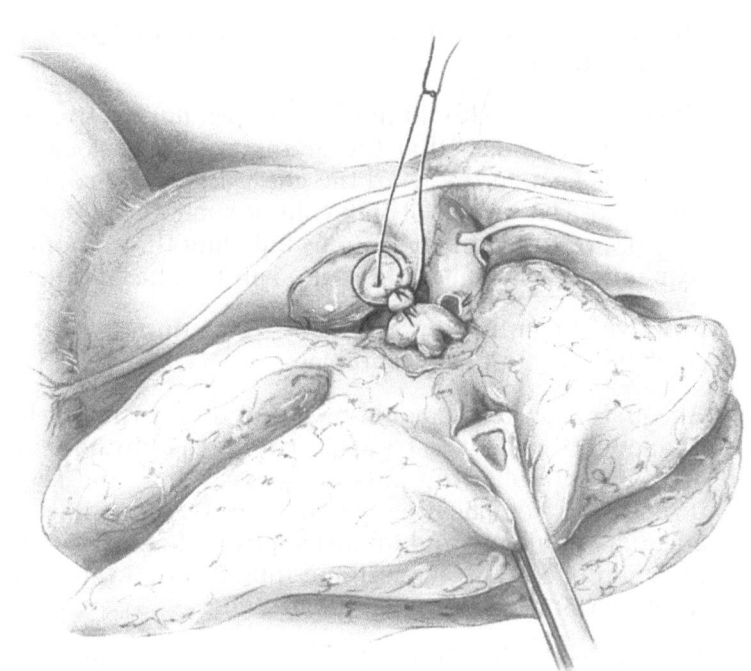

6 The previously tied left superior pulmonary vein is transfixed and tied and also secured distally.

7

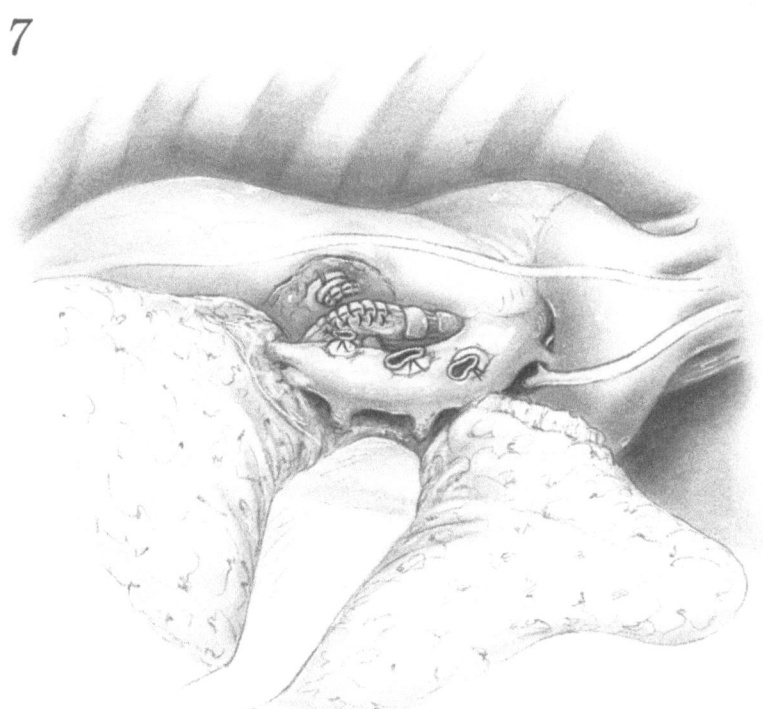

7 After the left superior pulmonary vein has been divided, the left upper lobe is removed. The left lower lobe is then allowed to expand to fill the left hemithorax.

The incision is closed in layers with anterior and posterior drainage tubes, with sideholes, extending up to the apex.

The chest drains should not be clamped during transport of the patient back to the ward, and care must be taken that the drains are not dislodged or kinked during movement. Once the patient is back in the ward the chest drains are connected to suction which must have careful control and be capable of high volume suction. Suction should be sufficient to maintain a negative pressure resulting in continuous bubbling throughout the respiratory cycle. Tubes are removed sequentially when all drainage and air leak has stopped.

Prophylactic antibiotics should be discontinued after 24 h. Antibiotics are thereafter only indicated for specific infective problems.

Adequate pain relief should be ensured to permit early and full movement of the shoulder and to allow the patient to co-operate with the physiotherapist in expectoration. Sputum problems are common following pulmonary resection, and if not dealt with promptly, will lead to life-threatening complications such as pulmonary infection. If sputum retention occurs despite adequate analgesia and intensive physiotherapy, suction bronchoscopy may be necessary. The insertion of a minitracheostomy tube through the cricothyroid membrane has largely replaced the performance of formal tracheostomy.

Cardiac dysrhythmias, particularly atrial tachycardias, are common following pulmonary resection, and prophylactic digoxin is often used in the elderly.

With the emphasis on early mobilisation, deep venous thrombosis and pulmonary embolism are now rarities and there is no evidence that low dose heparin is of any value.

11 Right Radical Pneumonectomy

Right pneumonectomy should only be performed when a lesser resection will not clear the pathological process. The commonest such indication in the western world is carcinoma of the bronchus. The tumour and involved lymph nodes must be confined to the lung, and lines of resection through vessels and bronchus should be clear of tumour. Radical pneumonectomy permits en bloc resection of the tumour with the superior mediastinal lymph nodes. The right lung is the larger of the two, and careful assessment of respiratory function is necessary pre-operatively. All patients should be instructed pre-operatively in the physiotherapy manoeuvres which will be undertaken post-operatively. When undertaken for pulmonary sepsis, pre-operative physiotherapy may produce a temporary but important improvement in the patient's condition and help minimise post-operative sputum difficulties. Prophylactic antibiotics commenced with the premedication and continued for 24 h have been shown to reduce the incidence of wound infection but will have no influence on the more serious problems of chest infection and infection of the pleural space.

An endobronchial tube passed by the anaesthetist will allow single lung ventilation. The collapse of the lung on the side of surgery will minimise the competing aims of surgeon and anaesthetist.

1

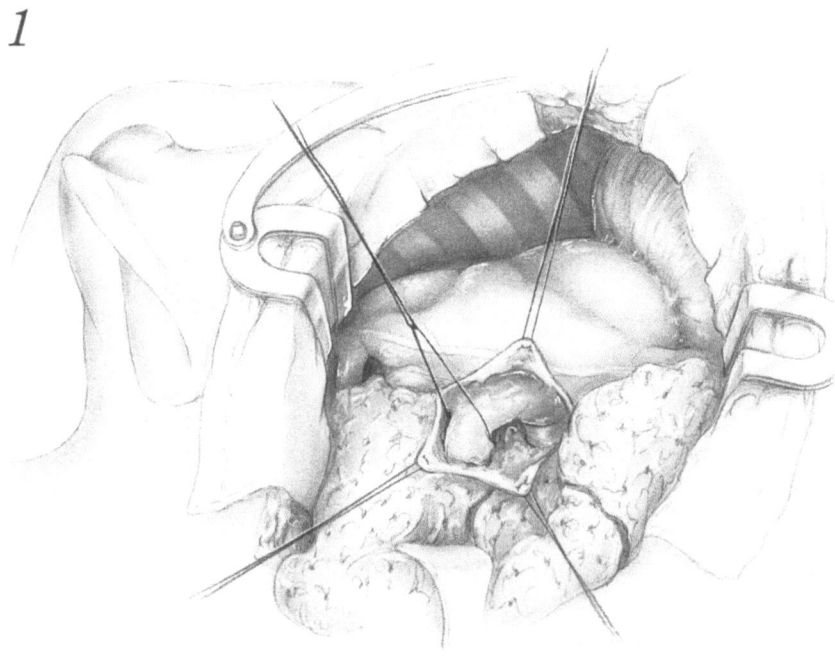

1 The pericardium is opened in front of the pulmonary veins (behind and parallel to the phrenic) to expose the two pulmonary veins. The superior pulmonary vein is surrounded with a ligature.

2

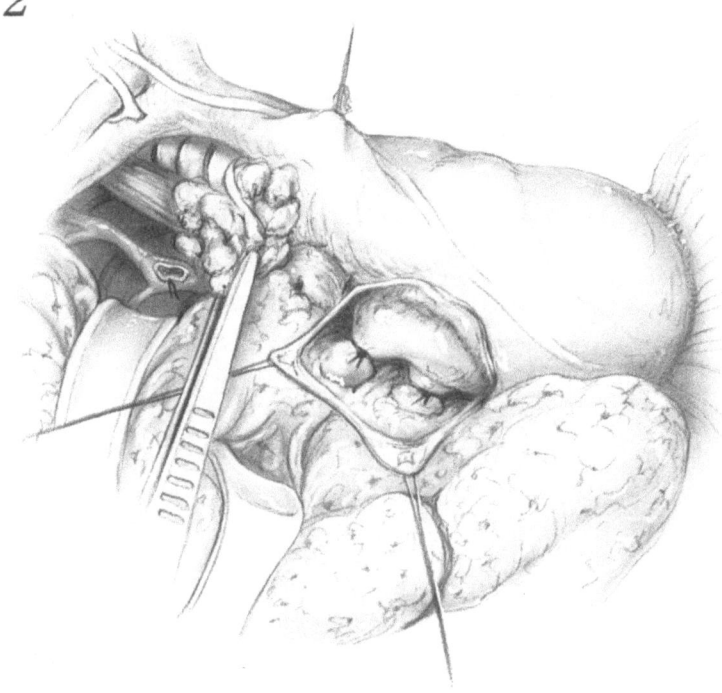

2 Both right pulmonary veins have been tied inside the pericardium.

3

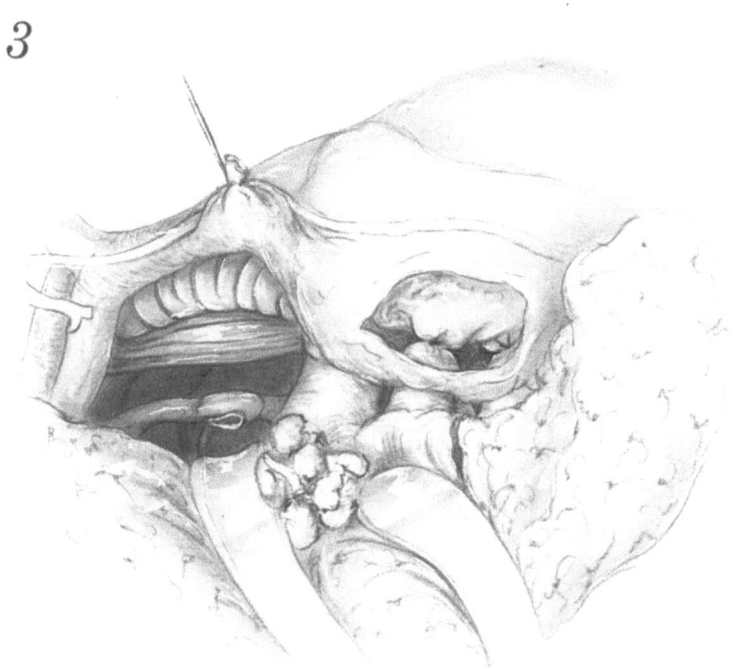

3 The superior mediastinal block dissection has been completed by dividing the azygos arch between ligatures, dividing the vagus below its recurrent branch and dissecting the fat and lymph nodes downwards towards the right pulmonary artery.

4

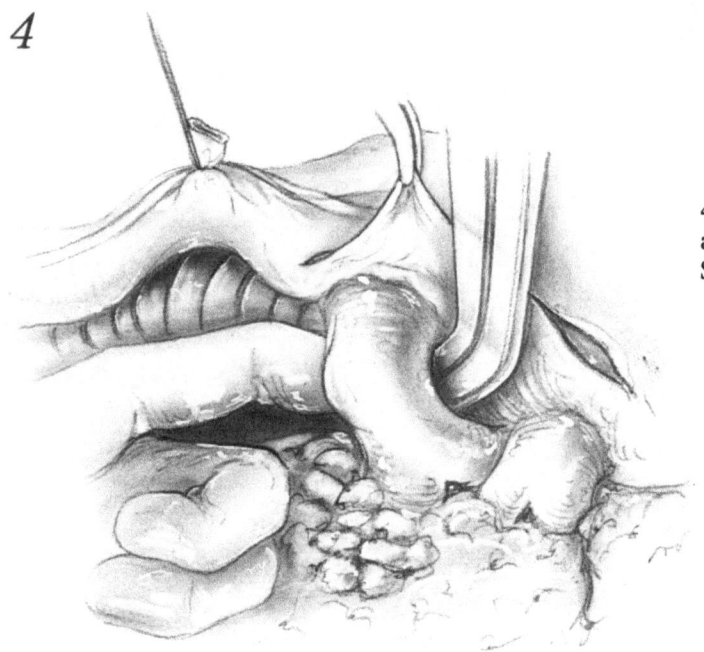

4 The right pulmonary artery is dissected out at its origin using the left index finger and a Semb dissection clamp.

5

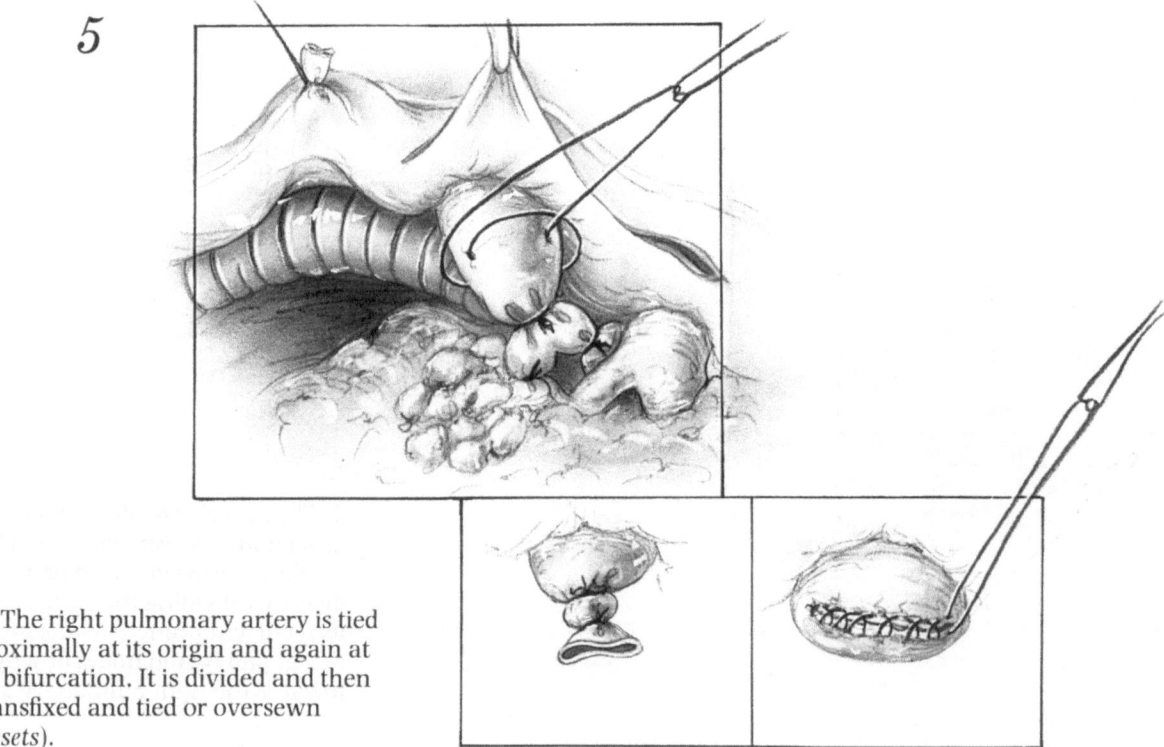

5 The right pulmonary artery is tied proximally at its origin and again at its bifurcation. It is divided and then transfixed and tied or oversewn (*insets*).

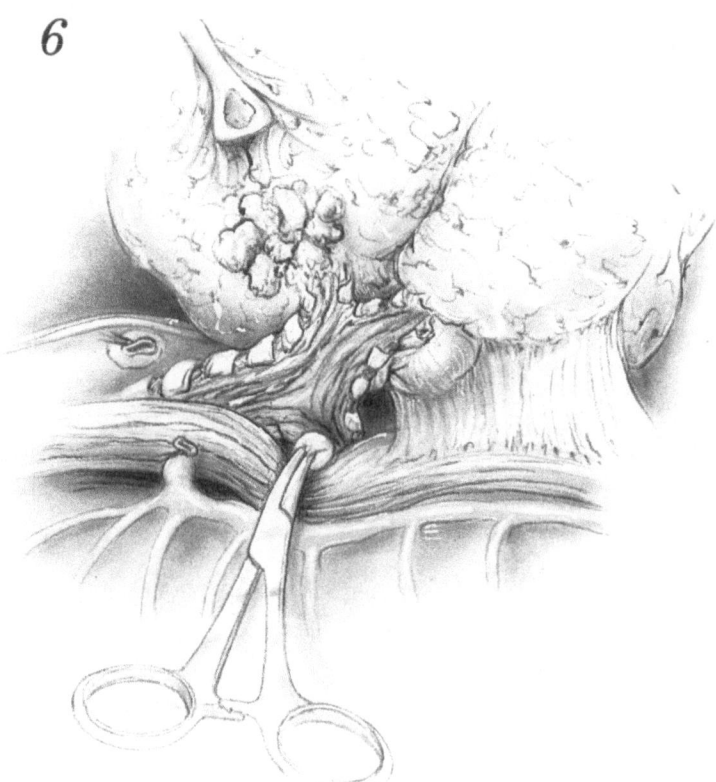

6 The right main bronchus is exposed by continuing the block dissection downwards in front of the oesophagus (retracted with a dissecting swab).

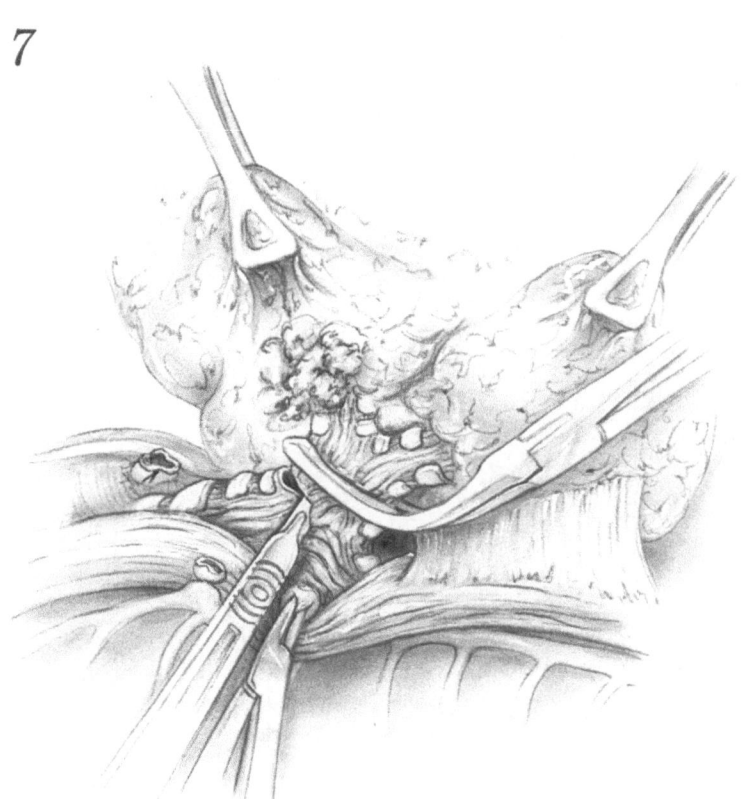

7 The right main bronchus is clamped distally and divided at its origin.

8

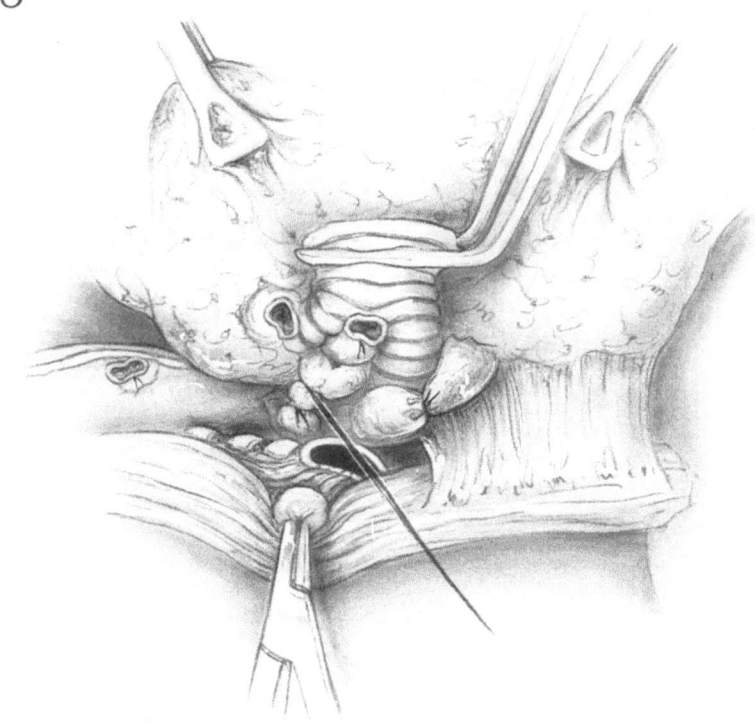

8 The previously tied pulmonary veins are secured distally, transfixed and tied *or* **9** they may be clamped distally, transfixed and tied and divided.

9

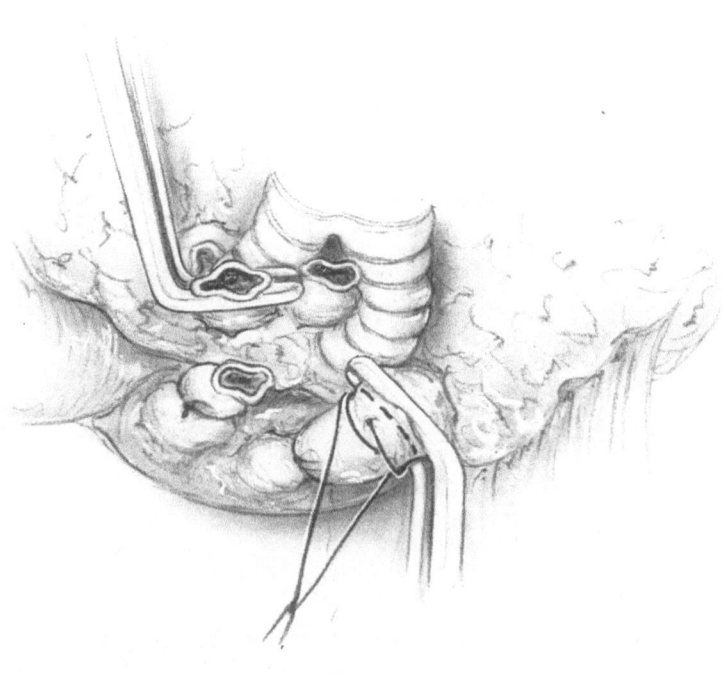

10

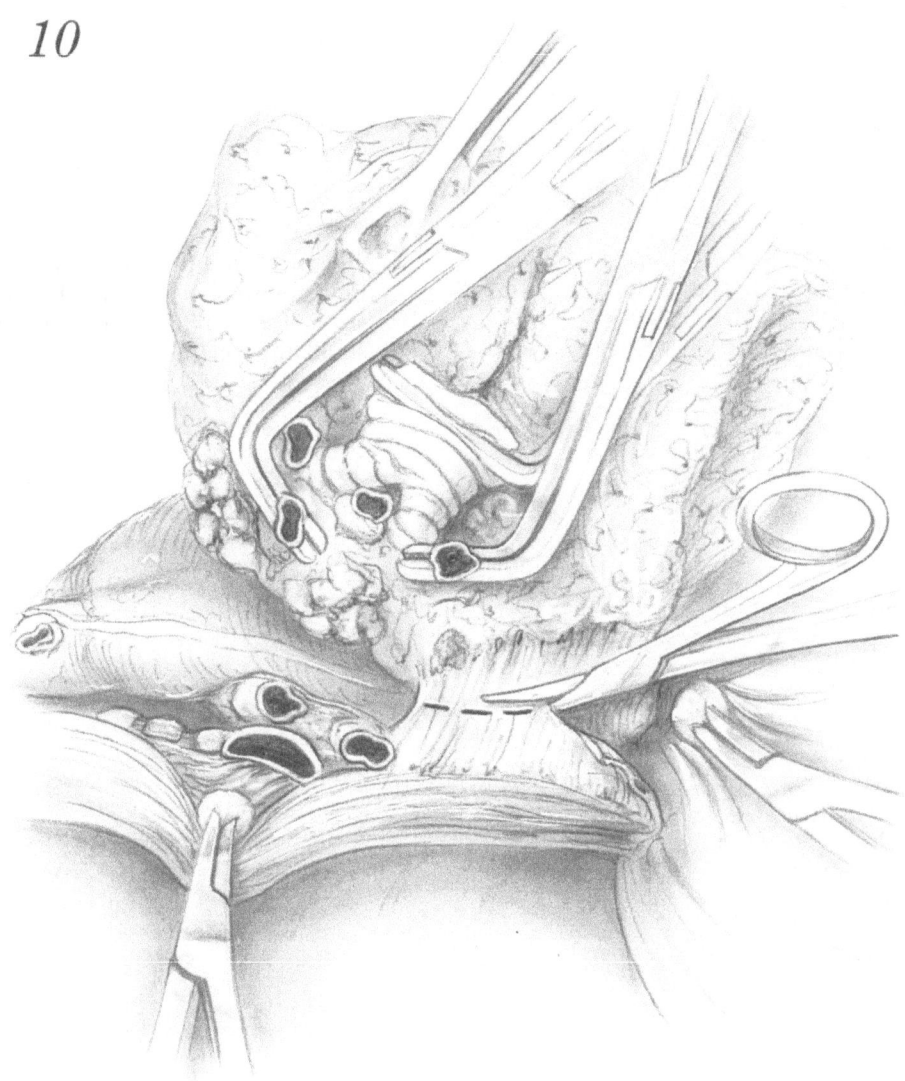

10 The inferior pulmonary ligament is divided, pushing the diaphragm down to gain exposure.

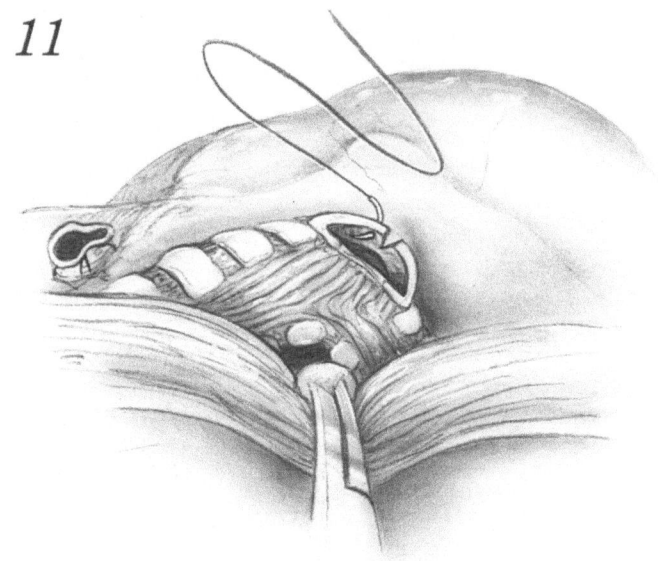

11 The right lung with all attached glands has been removed and the bronchial stump is closed (cartilage to cartilage by a small incision).

12a Bronchial closure is completed by a series of interrupted vertical mattress sutures **b** covered by a continuous over-and-over suture of 3-0 prolene.

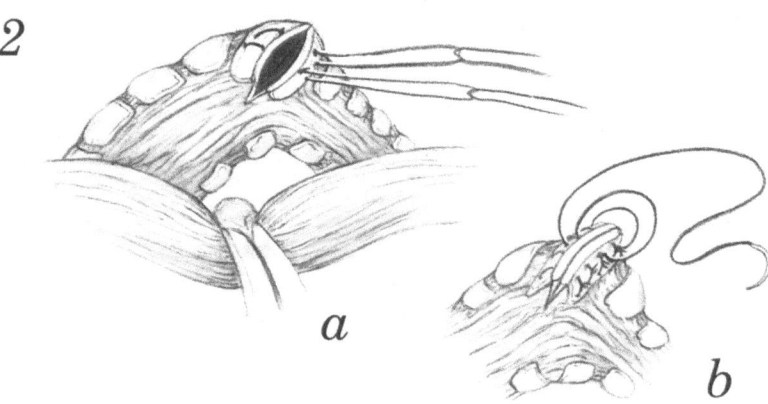

a

b

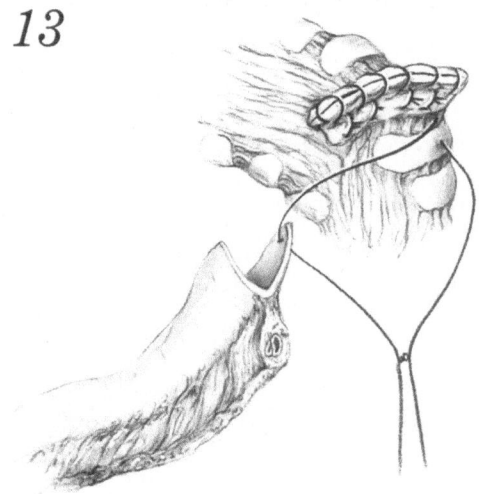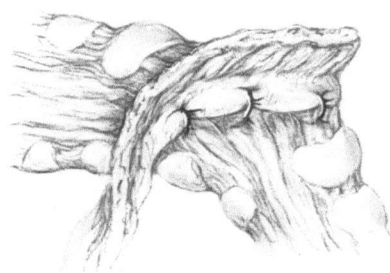

13 The bronchial suture line is covered by the previously prepared intercostal muscle bundle held in place by single sutures.

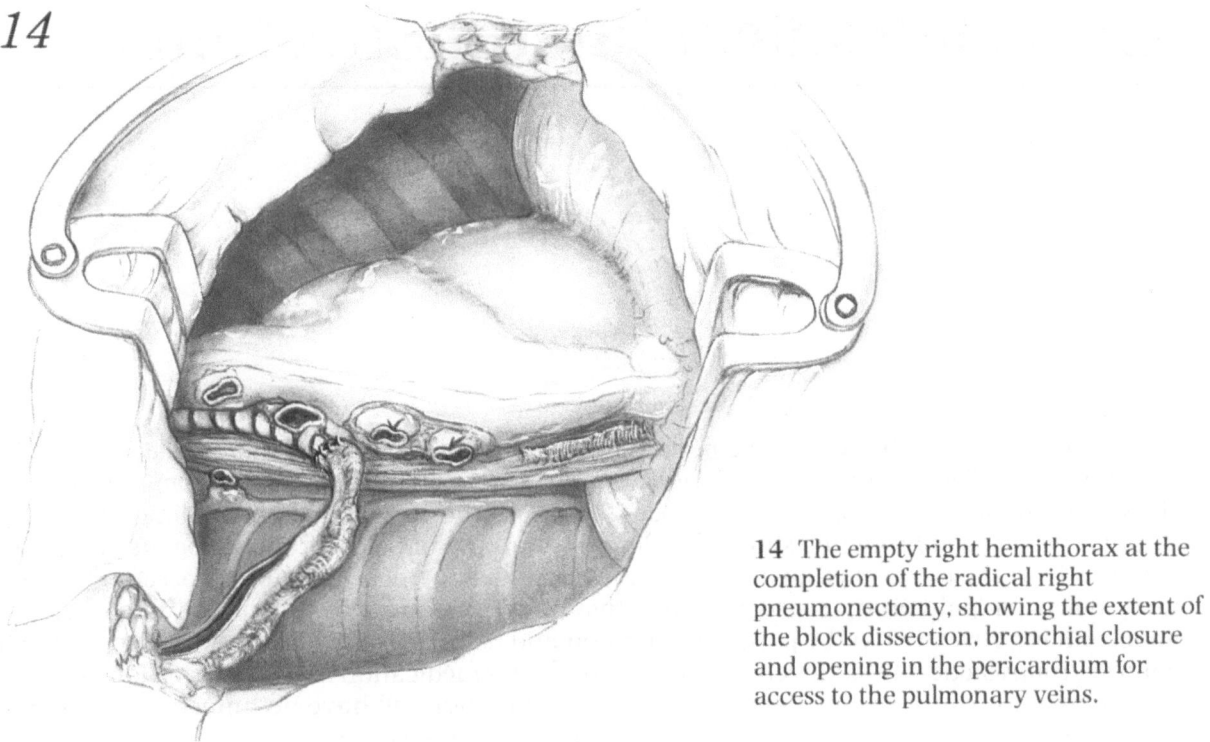

14 The empty right hemithorax at the completion of the radical right pneumonectomy, showing the extent of the block dissection, bronchial closure and opening in the pericardium for access to the pulmonary veins.

The incision is closed, placing in position one drainage tube without sideholes. The top of the tube should only be as high as the top of the right diaphragm. This tube is released for 1 min every hour and is removed after 24 h unless bleeding is excessive. Suction should never be applied to this drain. Before removal it may be used to correct any excessive mediastinal shift.

Prophylactic antibiotics should be discontinued after 24 h. Antibiotics are thereafter only indicated for specific infective problems. Adequate pain relief should be ensured to permit early and full movement of the shoulder and to allow the patient to co-operate with the physiotherapist in expectoration. Sputum problems are common following pulmonary resection, and if not dealt with promptly, will lead to life-threatening complications such as pulmonary infection. If sputum retention occurs despite adequate analgesia and intensive physiotherapy, suction bronchoscopy may be necessary. The insertion of a minitracheostomy tube through the cricothyroid membrane has largely replaced the performance of formal tracheostomy.

Cardiac dysrhythmias, particularly atrial tachycardias, are common following pulmonary resection, and prophylactic digoxin is often used in the elderly.

With the emphasis on early mobilisation, deep venous thrombosis and pulmonary embolism are now rarities and there is no evidence that low dose heparin is of any value.

12 Left Radical Pneumonectomy

Left pneumonectomy should only be performed when a lesser resection will not clear the pathological process. The commonest such indication in the western world is carcinoma of the bronchus. The tumour and involved lymph nodes must be confined to the lung, and lines of resection through vessels and bronchus should be clear of tumour. All patients should be instructed pre-operatively in the physiotherapy manoeuvres which will be undertaken post-operatively. When undertaken for pulmonary sepsis pre-operative physiotherapy may produce a temporary but important improvement in the patient's condition and help minimise post-operative sputum difficulties. Prophylactic antibiotics commenced with the premedication and continued for 24 h have been shown to reduce the incidence of wound infection but will have no influence on the more serious problems of chest infection and infection of the pleural space.

An endobronchial tube passed by the anaesthetist will allow single lung ventilation. The collapse of the lung on the side of surgery will minimise the competing aims of surgeon and anaesthetist.

1

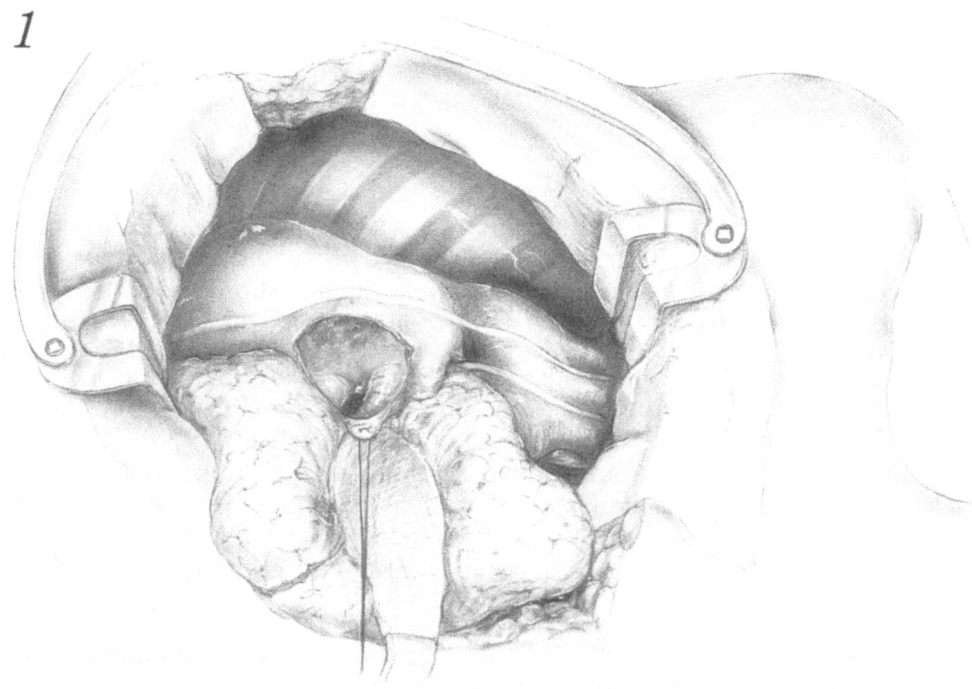

1 The left chest has been entered by stripping the lower border of the fifth rib. The left pulmonary veins are exposed by opening the pericardium immediately behind the phrenic nerve.

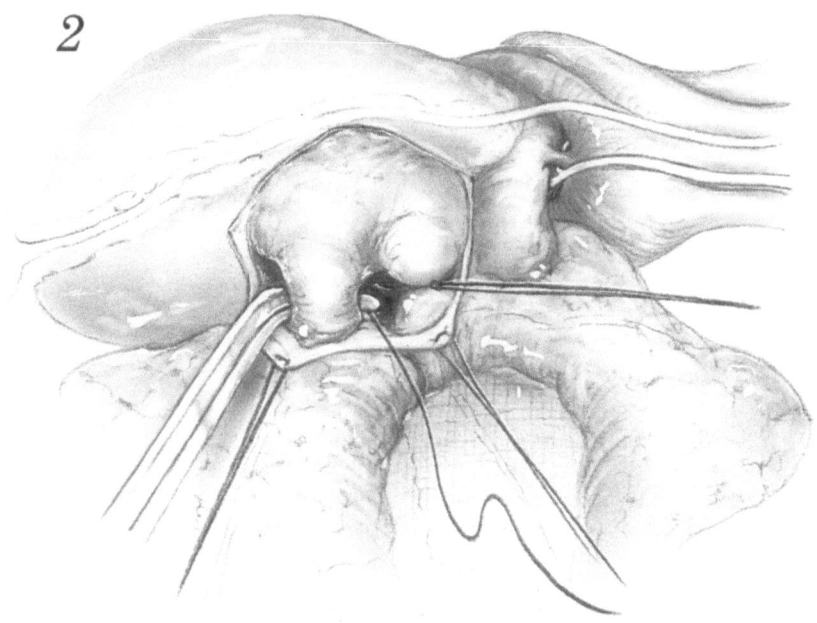

2 Both pulmonary veins are tied as a first step.

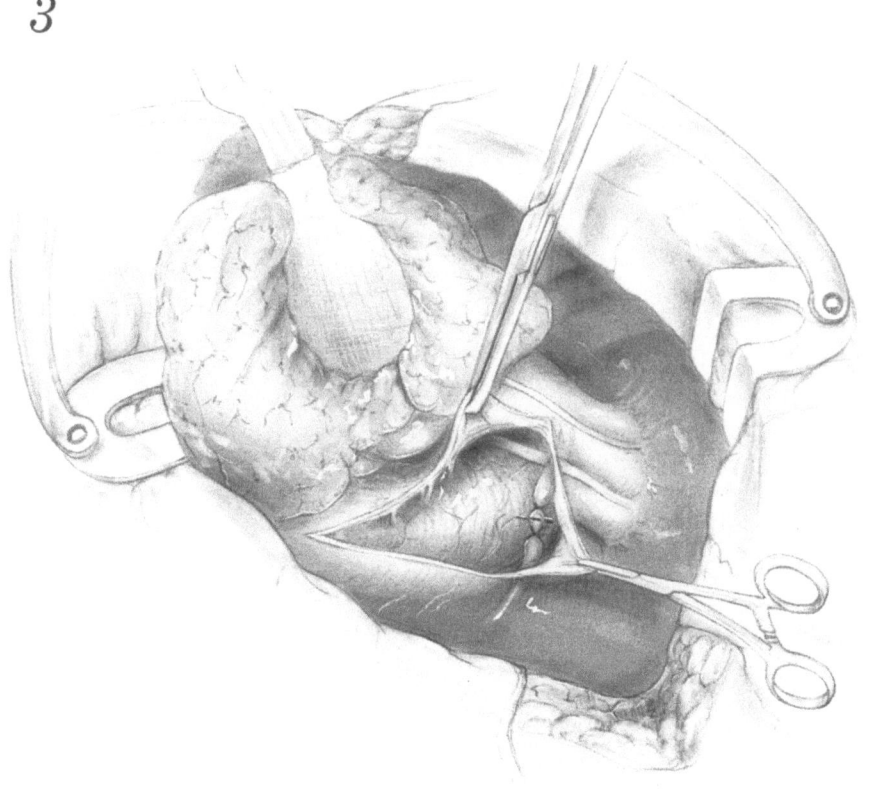

3 The fascia overlying the aorta is dissected and the superior intercostal vein is tied and divided.

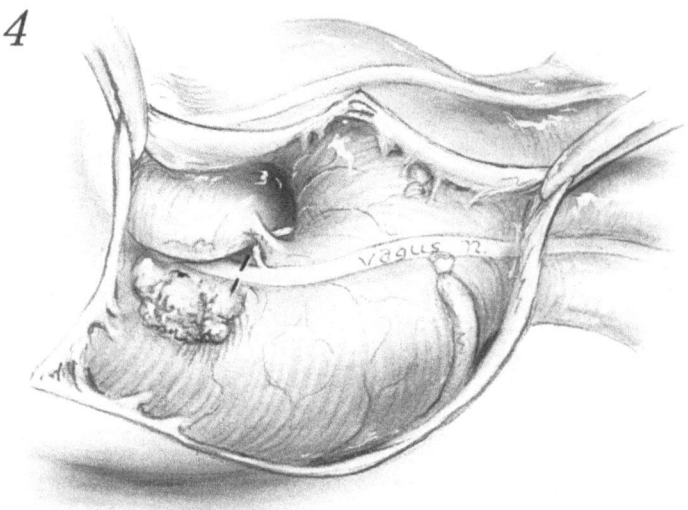

4 The fascia is reflected off the vagus, identifying its recurrent branch,

5 and the vagus is then divided below this level.

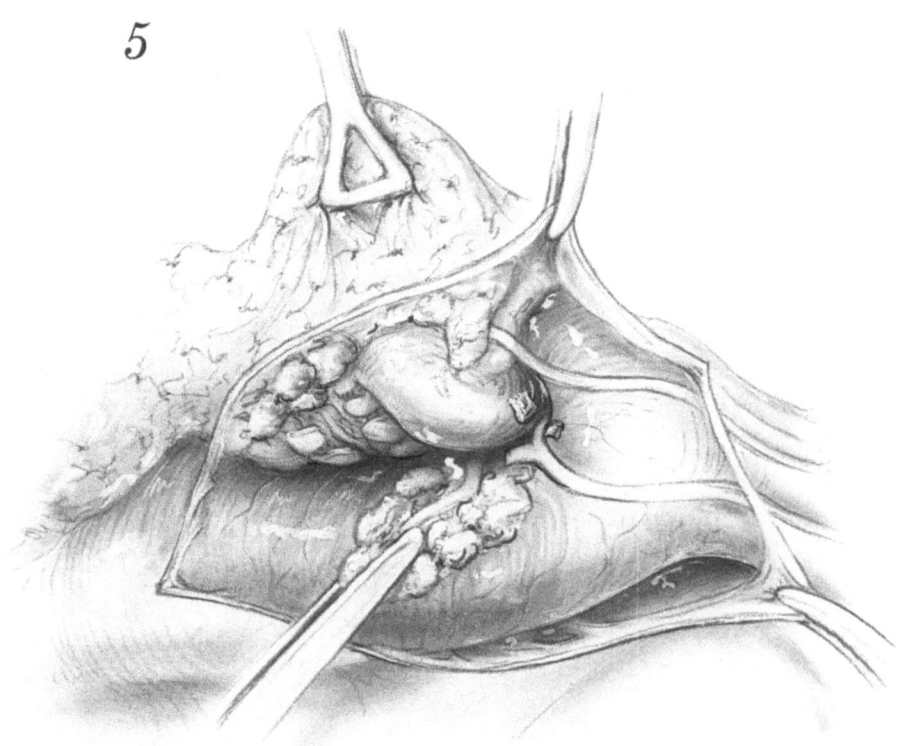

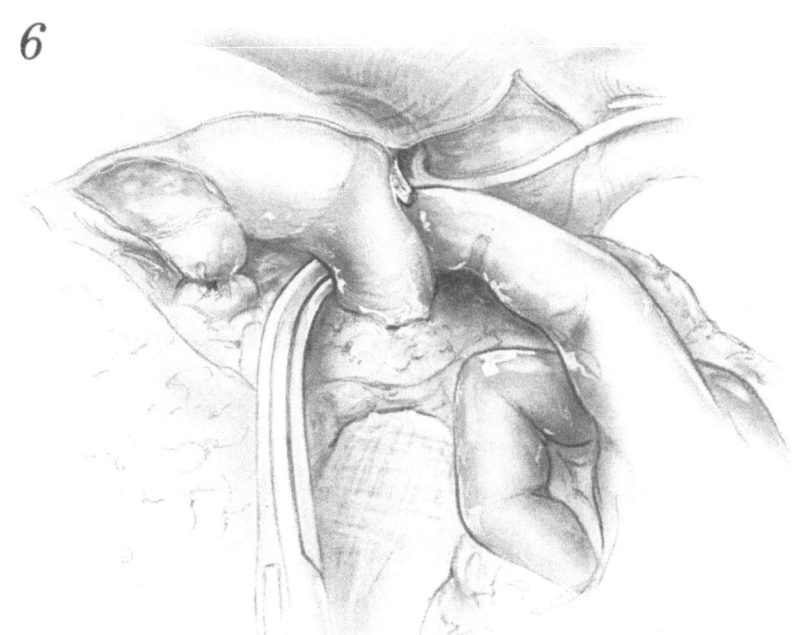

6 The left main pulmonary artery
is identified and dissected out with
blunt dissection and a Semb
clamp.

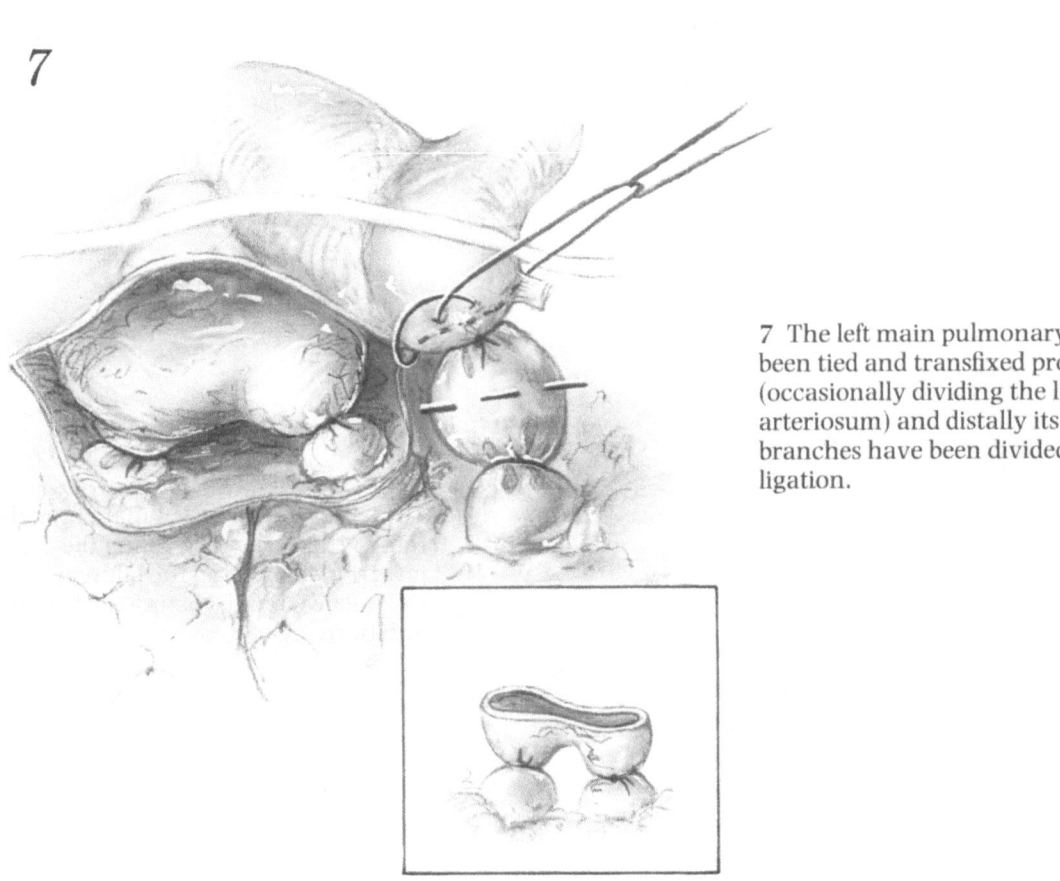

7 The left main pulmonary artery has
been tied and transfixed proximally
(occasionally dividing the ligamentum
arteriosum) and distally its first two
branches have been divided after
ligation.

8

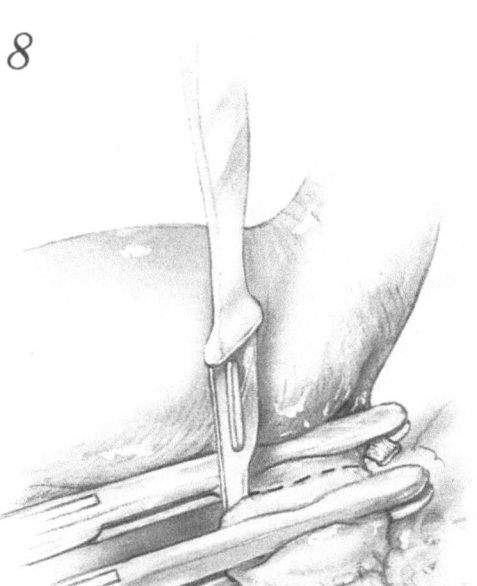

9

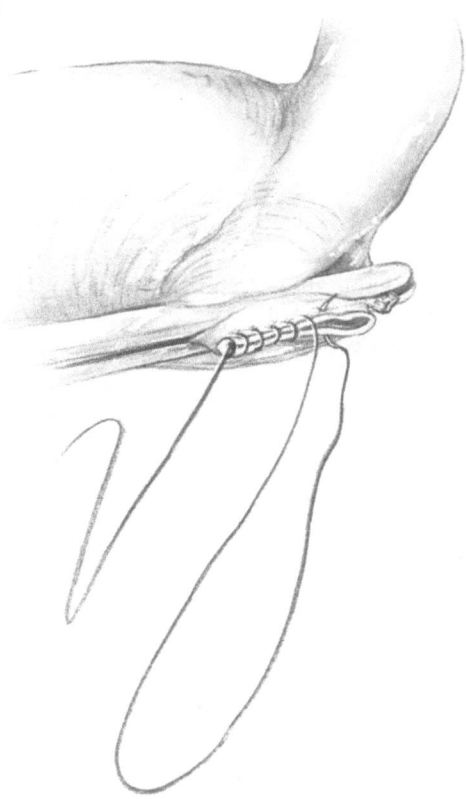

8 Alternatively, if there is insufficient length, the pulmonary artery may be divided between clamps,

9 and its central stump can then be oversewn.

10

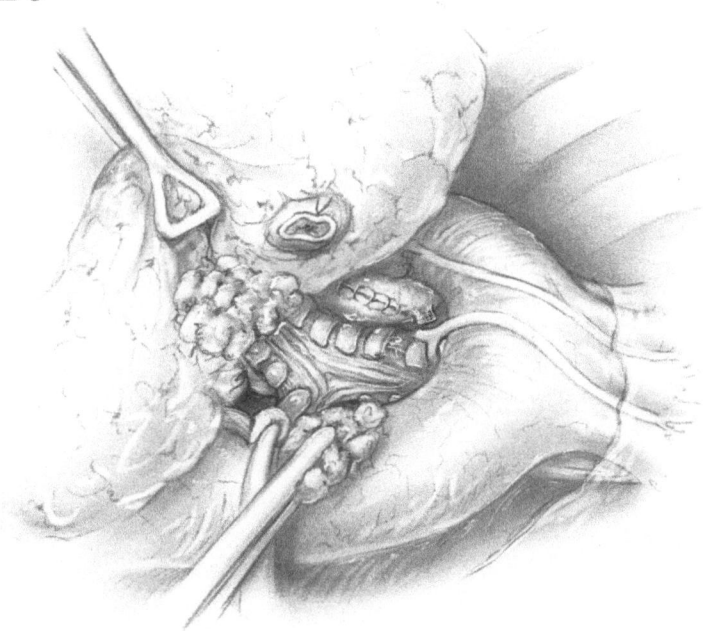

10 The origin of the left main bronchus is then exposed by retracting the aorta posteriorly, exposing the bifurcation of the trachea and retracting the left lung anteriorly.

11

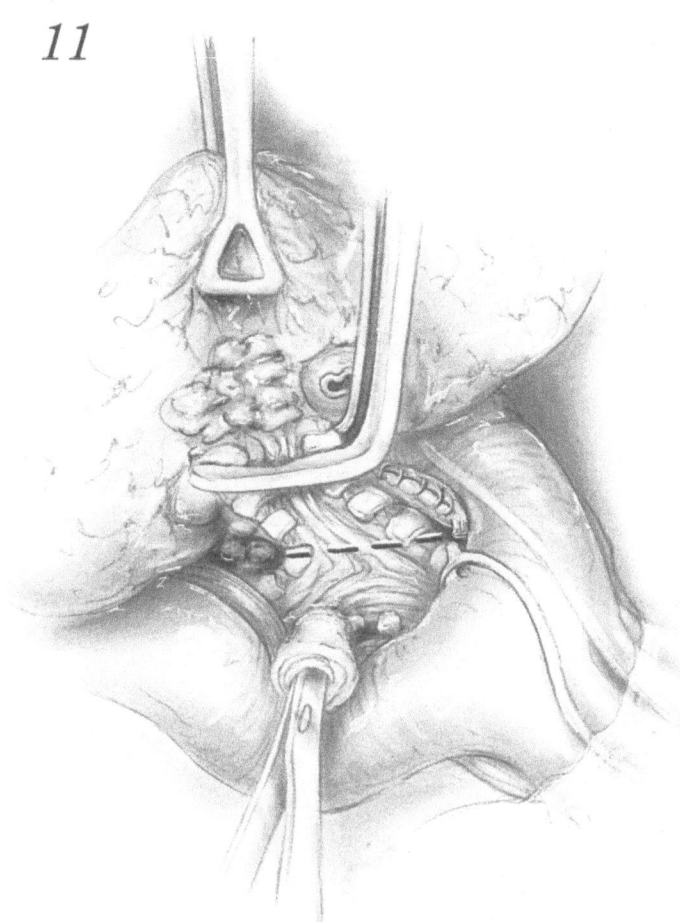

11 The left main bronchus is clamped and then divided obliquely.

12

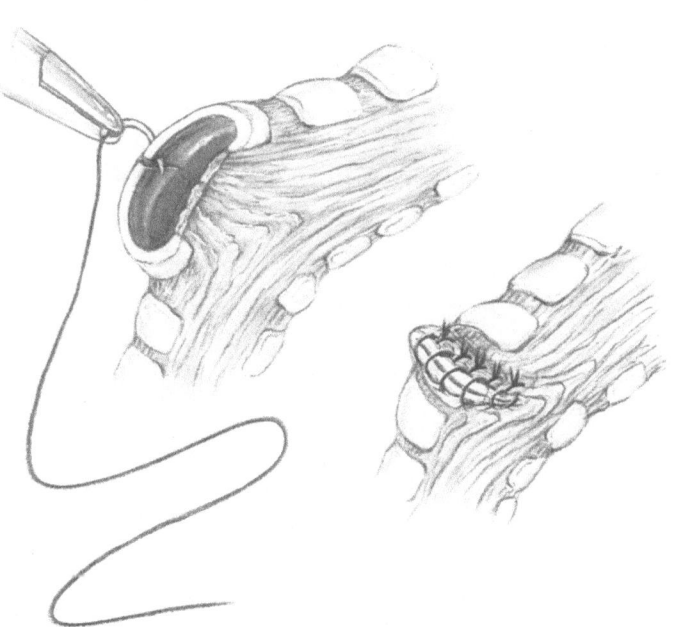

12 The bronchial stump is closed transversely so as to appose the two halves of the cartilaginous ring, having incised this ring anteriorly so as to allow the closure to be carried out without tension. This is performed in the usual way with interrupted vertical mattress sutures covered by a continuous stitch.

13

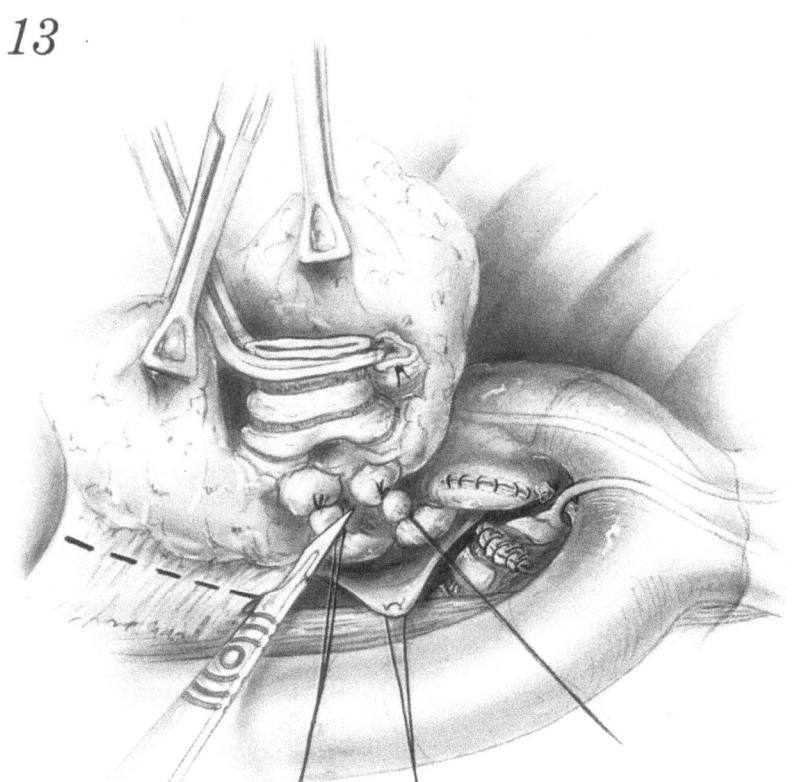

13 The two previously ligated pulmonary veins are tied distally and divided and transfixed.

14

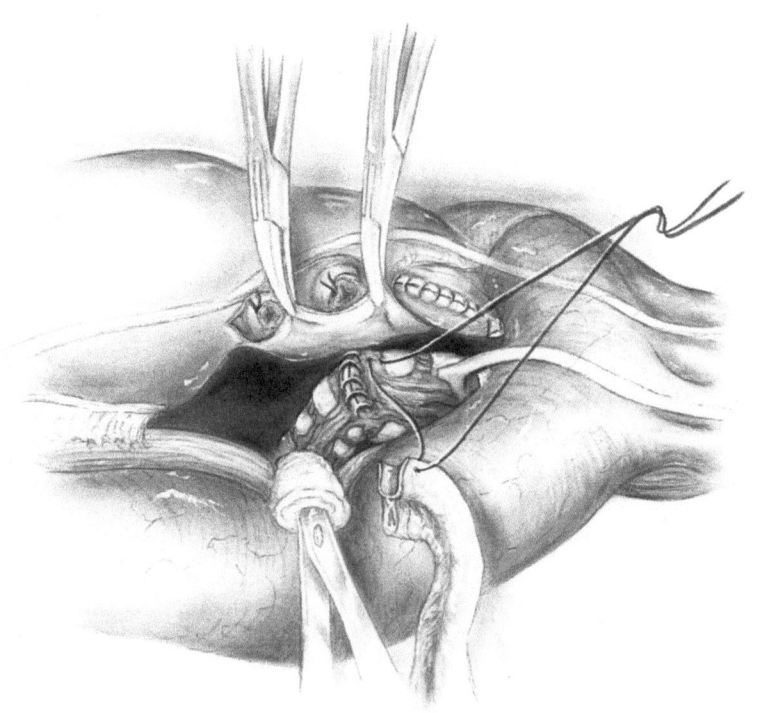

14 By retracting the posterior pericardium forwards, good access is obtained to the bronchial stump.

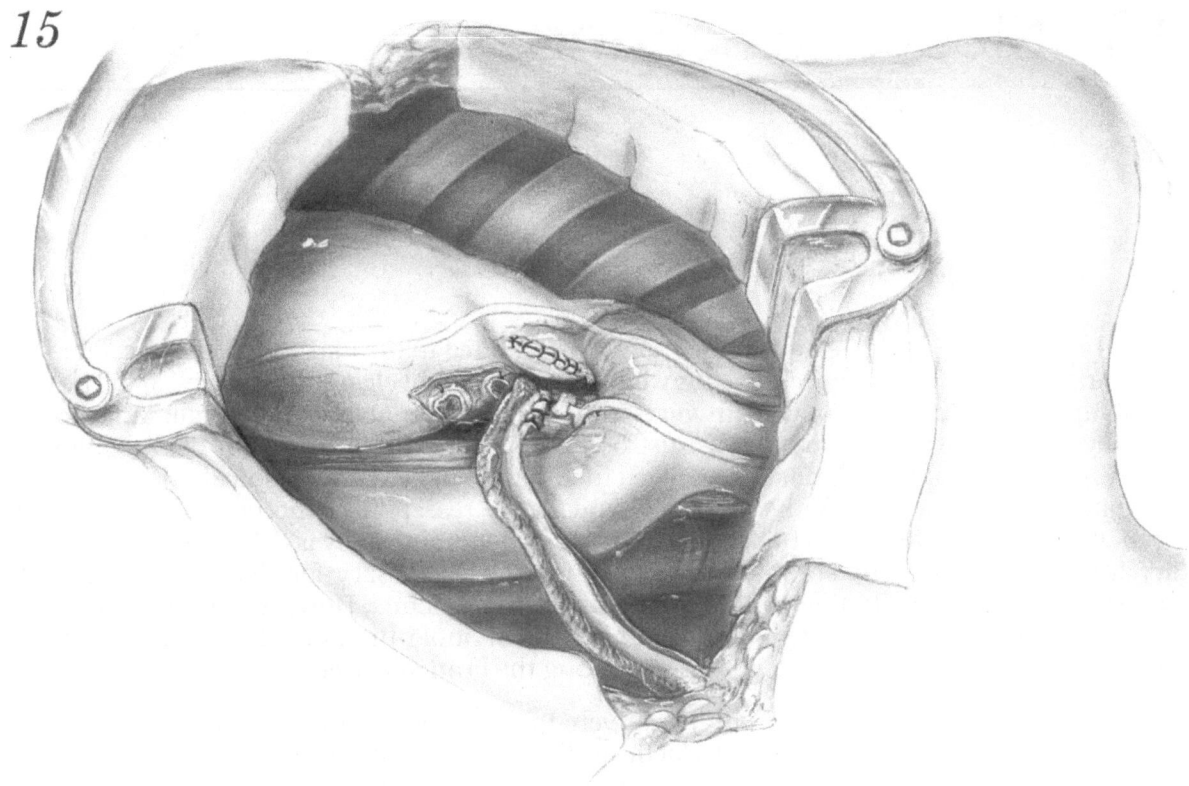

15 The previously prepared intercostal muscle bundle is attached with single stitches. General view of completed pneumonectomy showing the sutured central stump of the left main pulmonary artery, the bronchial stump covered by the intercostal muscle bundle, and the stumps of the two left pulmonary veins.

The incision is closed, placing in position one drainage tube without sideholes. The top of the tube should only be as high as the top of the left diaphragm. This tube is released for 1 min every hour and is removed after 24 h unless bleeding is excessive. Suction should never be applied to this drain.

Prophylactic antibiotics should be discontinued after 24 h. Antibiotics are thereafter only indicated for specific infective problems. Adequate pain relief should be ensured to permit early and full movement of the shoulder and to allow the patient to co-operate with the physiotherapist in expectoration. Sputum problems are common following pulmonary resection, and if not dealt with promptly, will lead to life-threatening complications such as pulmonary infection. If sputum retention occurs despite adequate analgesia and intensive physiotherapy, suction bronchoscopy may be necessary, and the insertion of a minitracheostomy tube through the cricothyroid membrane has largely replaced the performance of formal tracheostomy.

Cardiac dysrhythmias, particularly atrial tachycardias, are common following pulmonary resection, and prophylactic digoxin is often used in the elderly.

With the emphasis on early mobilisation, deep venous thrombosis and pulmonary embolism are now rarities and there is no evidence that low dose heparin is of any value.

13 Sleeve Resection

A sleeve resection is indicated when the tumour is confined to the upper lobe, the vascular structures are accessible as for upper lobectomy but wider bronchial clearance is necessary. The origin of the upper lobe bronchus may be involved, but the main bronchus at its origin and the intermediate bronchus at its termination must be clear of infiltration. Invasion of the pulmonary artery at this level or the presence of involved hilar lymph nodes contra-indicate sleeve resection. Although sleeve resection of the bronchus and sleeve resection of the pulmonary artery has been undertaken, disastrous fistulae may occur, and pneumonectomy is to be preferred if pulmonary function permits. The strict anatomical restrictions necessary for sleeve resection will be encountered from time to time with carcinoma of the bronchus. However, bronchoplastic procedures are of particular value when dealing with carcinoid tumours. These tumours tend to arise from carinae but have limited extension along the bronchial tree.

All patients should be instructed pre-operatively in the physiotherapy manoeuvres which will be undertaken post-operatively. Prophylactic antibiotics commenced with the premedication and continued for 24 h have been shown to reduce the incidence of wound infection but will have no influence on the more serious problems of chest infection and infection of the pleural space.

Right Upper Sleeve Resection

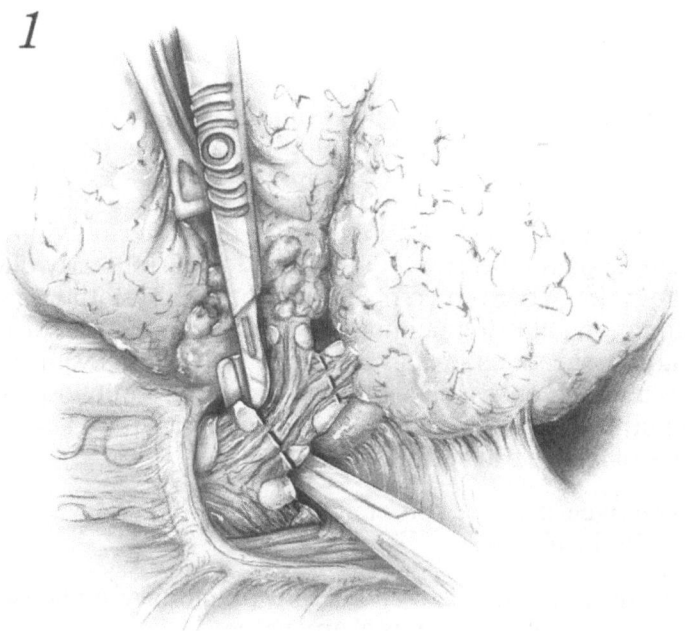

1 The branches of the pulmonary artery to the right upper lobe have been divided as for a right upper lobectomy (Chap. 5, Fig. 4). The origin of the right upper lobe bronchus is exposed and the right main bronchus is divided proximally, close to its origin, and distally just above the take-off of the apical lower bronchus at the back and the middle lobe bronchus in front (*dotted lines*).

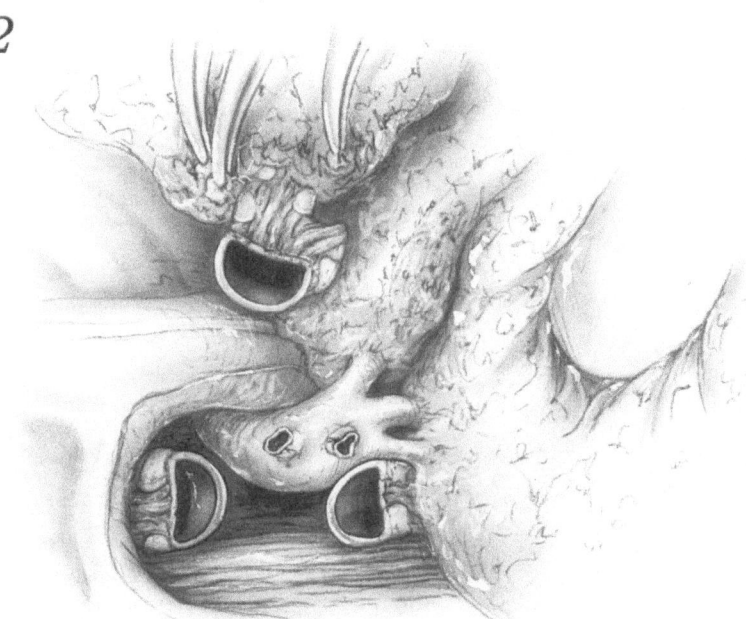

2 The segment of main bronchus with the origin of the upper lobe bronchus, the upper lobe and all attached lymph nodes, is removed. The superior pulmonary vein, exclusive of its middle lobe tributary, will have been tied and divided, as for a standard right upper lobectomy (see Chap. 5, Fig. 7).

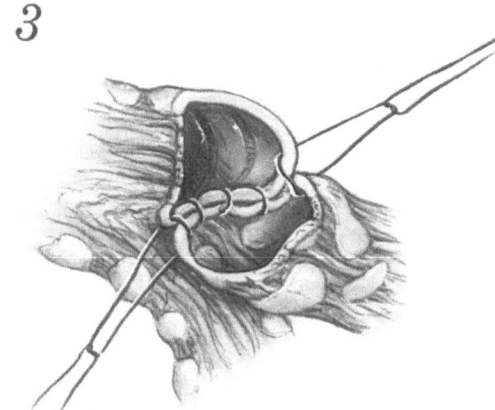

3 The two cut ends of the bronchus are anastomosed using interrupted monofilament sutures, starting at the deep edge and encircling one cartilage ring at each cut end. The membranous part of the bronchus is sutured last.

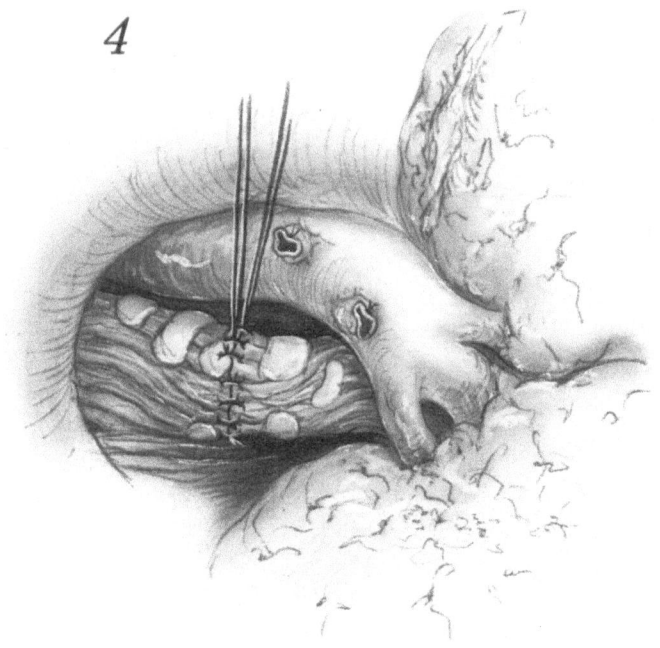

4 The completed anastomosis now allows the middle and lower lobes to be ventilated by the anaesthetist and the anastomosis is checked for airleaks. The chest is then closed routinely with two drainage tubes (see Chap. 5, Fig. 11).

5

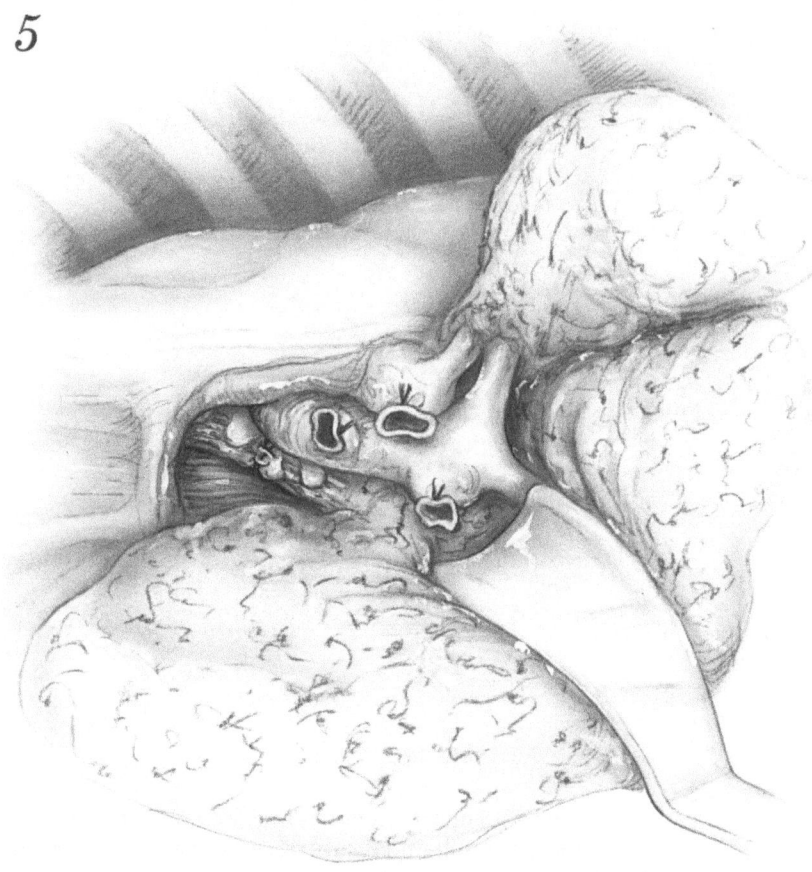

5 The close proximity of the
pulmonary artery and its
branches to the bronchial
anastomosis is shown. The tied
superior pulmonary vein with
its venous middle lobe
tributary is shown in front.

Left Upper Sleeve Resection

6 The branches of the pulmonary artery to the upper lobe have been tied and divided as for a standard left upper lobectomy (see Chap. 10, Figs. 4,5). The left pulmonary artery is retracted forwards and the origin of the left upper lobe bronchus is exposed. The lines of division of the main bronchus are shown: note that the lower line of division has to be oblique so as to spare the apical lower bronchus, which comes off virtually at the same level as the left upper lobe bronchus.

6

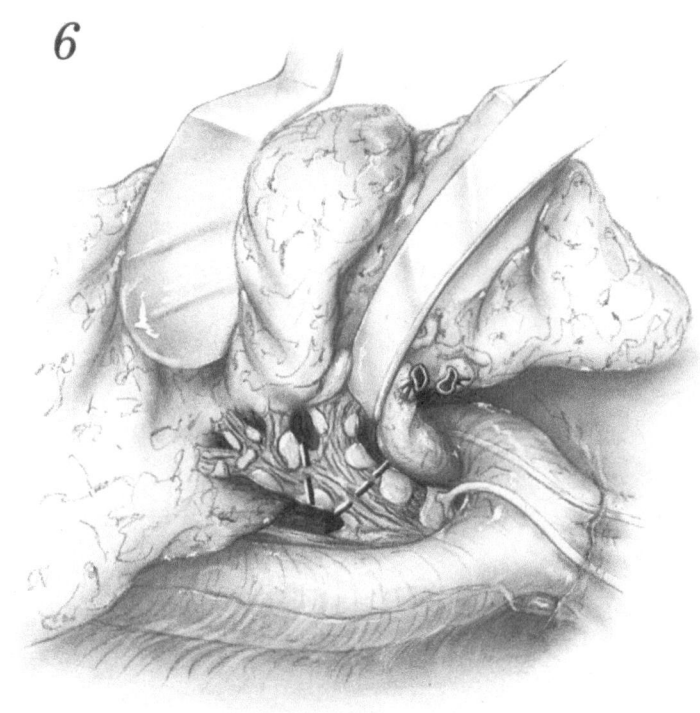

7

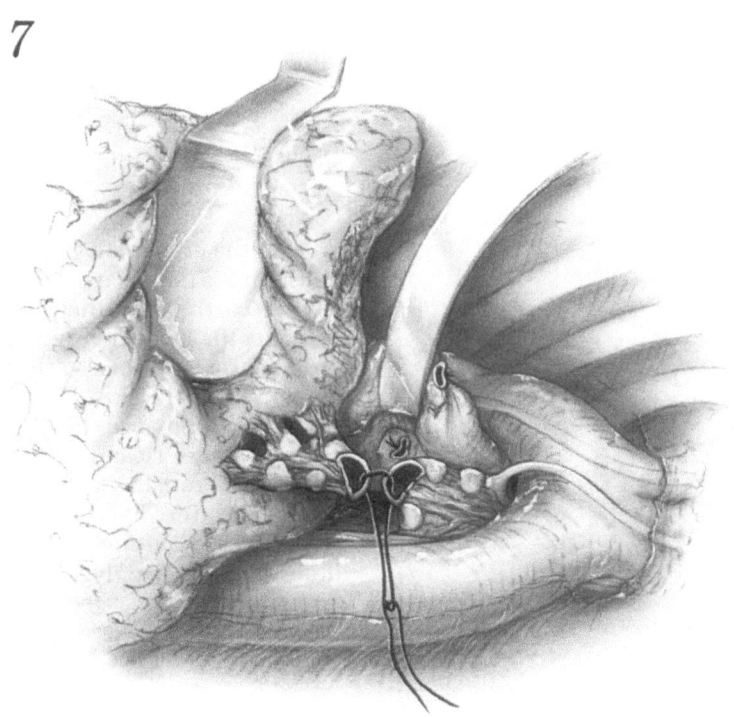

7 After the upper lobe has been removed (cf. Fig. 2) the lower lobe bronchus is anastomosed to the cut end of the main bronchus with interrupted monofilament suture, starting at the deep (anterior) edge and encircling one cartilage ring at each cut end. The membranous part is sutured last. The left pulmonary artery is retracted anteriorly to facilitate the bronchial anastomosis.

8

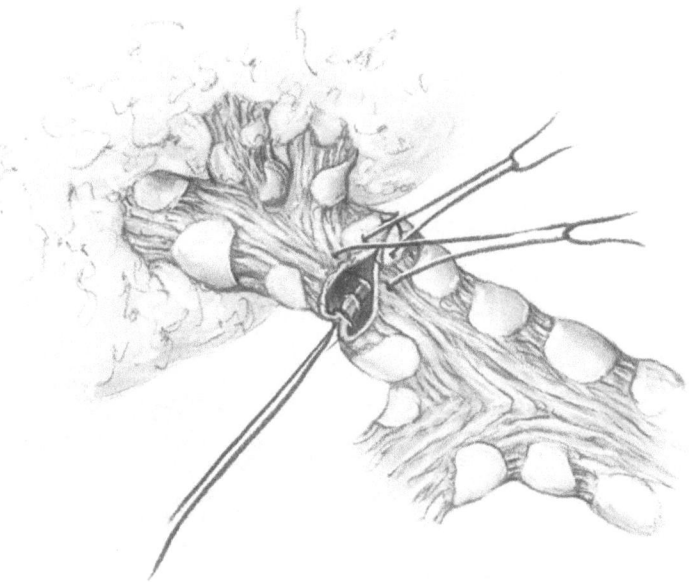

8 The bronchial anastomosis has almost been completed.

9

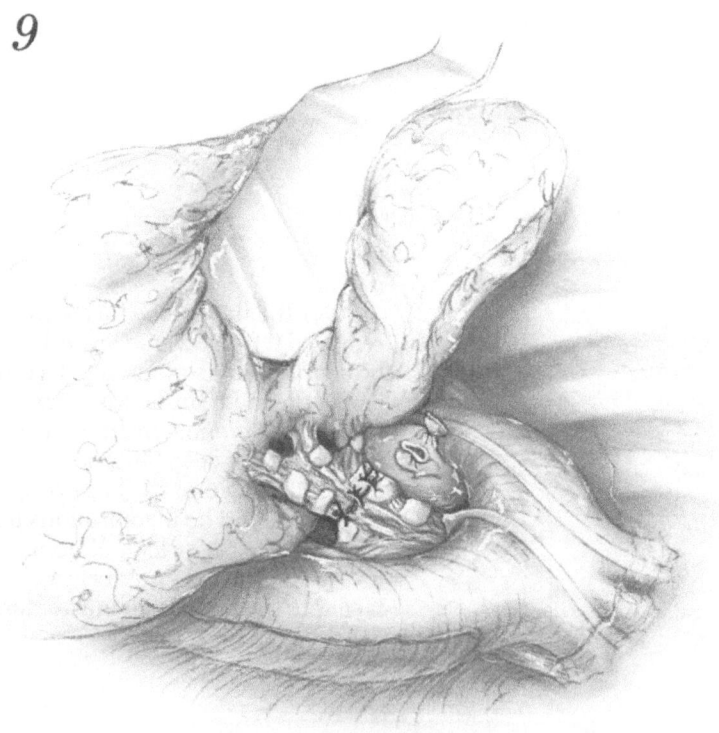

9 After the bronchial anastomosis has been completed, the anaesthetist can ventilate the lower lobe and the bronchial suture line is tested for airleak. (Note the close relationship between the pulmonary artery and its tied upper lobe branches to the bronchial suture line.) The chest is then closed routinely with two drains (see Chap. 5, Fig. 11).

Reverse Sleeve Resection—Right

10

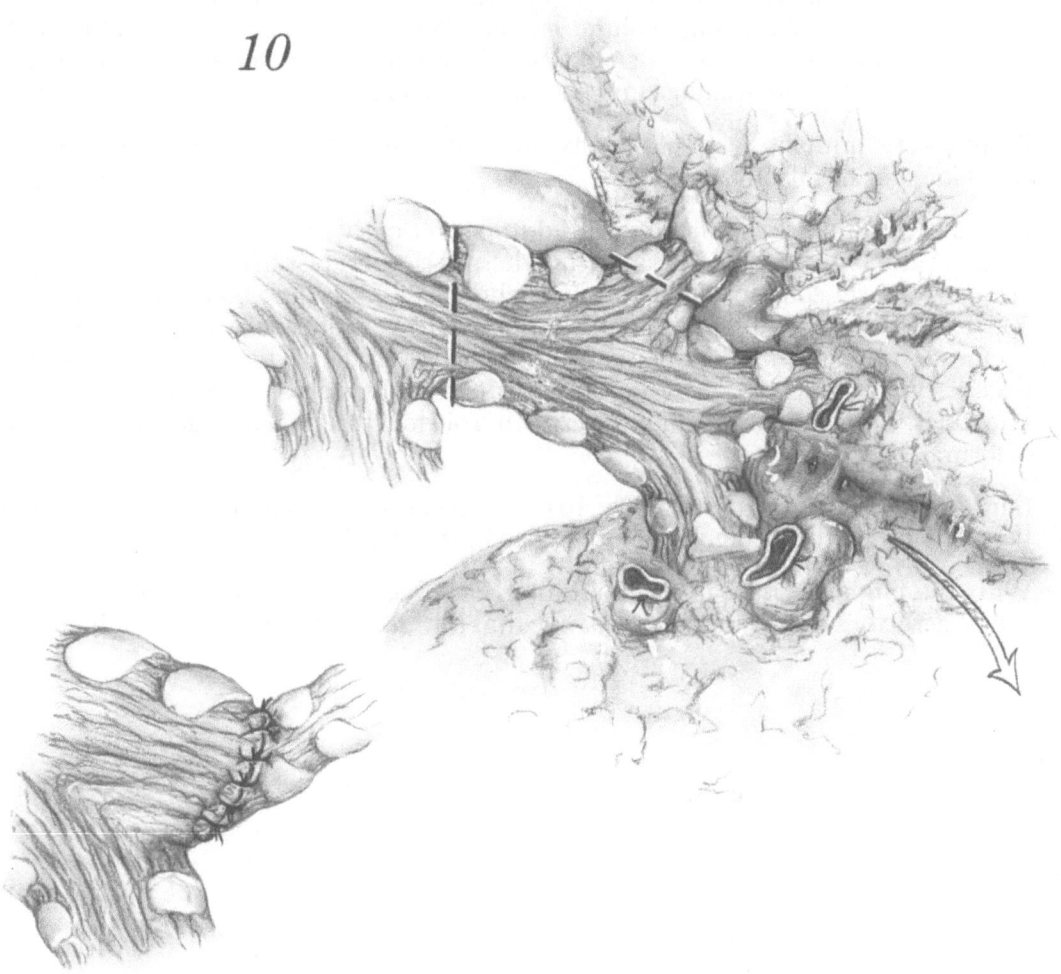

10 In this procedure the vessels to and from the right middle and lower lobes are dealt with as for a right middle and lower lobectomy (see Chap. 8, Fig. 3). The right main bronchus is divided at its origin and the right upper lobe bronchus is cut off the main bronchus as shown. The middle and lower lobes are removed and the right upper lobe bronchus is anastomosed to the origin of the main bronchus (*inset*). A similar procedure can be performed on the left side.

The incision is closed in layers with three drainage tubes with sideholes extending up to the apex. These chest drains should not be clamped during transport of the patient back to the ward and care must be taken that the drains are not dislodged or kinked during movement. Once the patient is back in the ward the chest drains are connected to suction which must have careful control and be capable of high volume suction. Suction should be sufficient to maintain a negative pressure resulting in continuous bubbling throughout the respiratory cycle. Tubes are removed sequentially when all drainage and air leak has stopped.

Prophylactic antibiotics should be discontinued after 24 h. Antibiotics are thereafter only indicated for specific infective problems.

Adequate pain relief should be ensured to permit early and full movement of the shoulder and to allow the patient to co-operate with the physiotherapist in expectoration. Sputum problems are particularly common following bronchoplastic procedures, and if not dealt with promptly, will lead to life-threatening complications such as pulmonary infection. If sputum retention occurs despite adequate analgesia and intensive physiotherapy, suction bronchoscopy may be necessary, care being taken not to disrupt the bronchial anastomosis. The insertion of a minitracheostomy tube through the cricothyroid membrane has largely replaced the performance of formal tracheostomy.

Cardiac dysrhythmias, particularly atrial tachycardias, are common following pulmonary resection, and prophylactic digoxin is often used in the elderly.

With the emphasis on early mobilisation, deep venous thrombosis and pulmonary embolism are now rarities and there is no evidence that low dose heparin is of any value.

14 Empyema—Decortication

Decortication or excision of an empyema is indicated when conservative means have failed. The empyema is usually preceded by an infected effusion which separates the parietal and visceral layers of the pleura. With chronicity the fluid becomes thicker and concentric lamellae of fibrous tissue are laid down, lining the pleural cavity and producing a parietal cortex covering the chest wall, diaphragm and mediastinum, and the visceral cortex covering the lung surface. In removing the empyema, the parietal cortex may be mobilised more easily by sacrificing the parietal pleura and dissecting the extrapleural plane. Once this has been achieved, however, further dissection requires the removal of the cortex covering the diaphragm and the lung, preserving the underlying pleura. Decortication is a major operation, being bloody and often tedious, and is not suitable for frail elderly patients. Its success relies on the underlying lung expanding to fill the hemithorax and this will depend upon the surgeon's ability to remove the cortex without too many breaches in the visceral pleura, and assumes that the underlying lung has recovered from the infective process and resumed its normal compliance. The timing of this operation in the infective process is therefore crucial, and this will vary depending on the underlying disease process. If portions of the lung are irreversibly damaged, decortication may be coupled with pulmonary resection. In young fit patients, decortication may be undertaken immediately the diagnosis is made, but in older patients a period of open drainage will improve the patient's suitability for operation and allow recovery from the infective process.

All patients should be instructed pre-operatively in the physiotherapy manoeuvres which will be undertaken post-operatively, and this may produce a temporary but important improvement in the patient's condition and help minimise post-operative sputum difficulties. Prophylactic antibiotics commenced with the premedication and continued for 24 h have been shown to reduce the incidence of wound infection, but will have no influence on the more serious problems of chest infection and infection of the pleural space.

An endobronchial tube passed by the anaesthetist will allow single lung ventilation. The collapse of the lung on the side of surgery will minimise the competing aims of surgeon and anaesthetist.

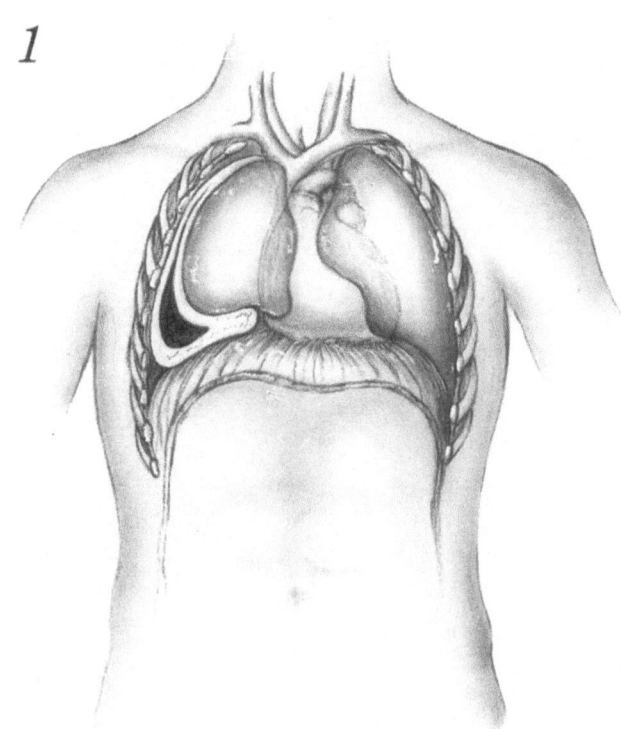

1 General view of the disposition of a right empyema.

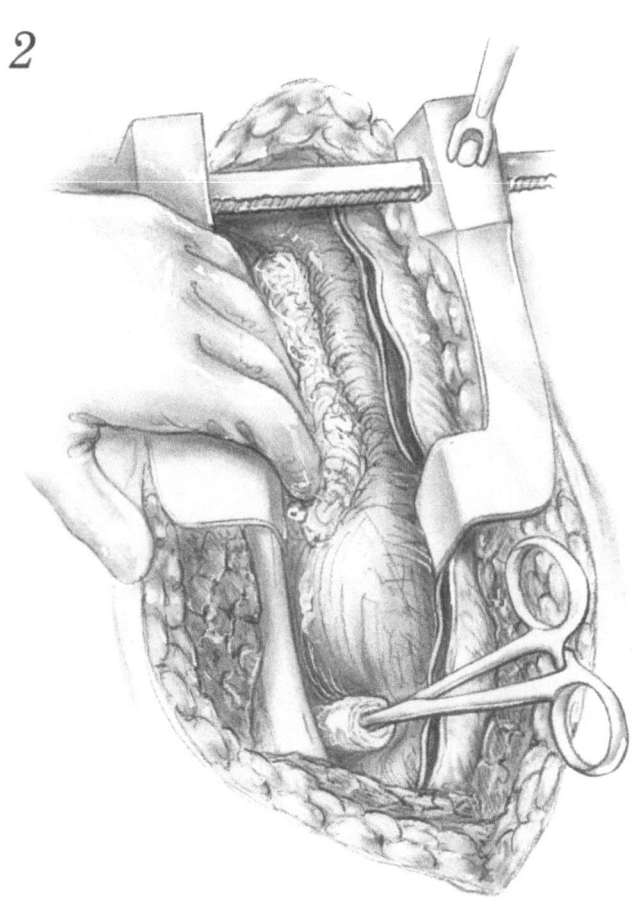

2 The subcostal incision can only be deepened gradually by blunt and sharp dissection.

3

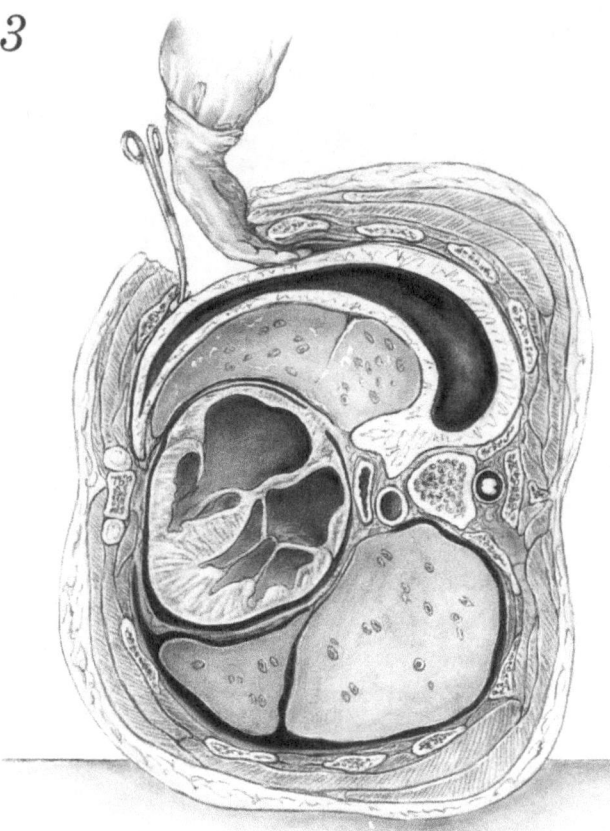

3 Technique of freeing the parietal layer of the empyema from the chest wall.

4

4 After sufficient freeing has been achieved, the chest can be widely opened and the cortex of the empyema dissected off the underlying lung.

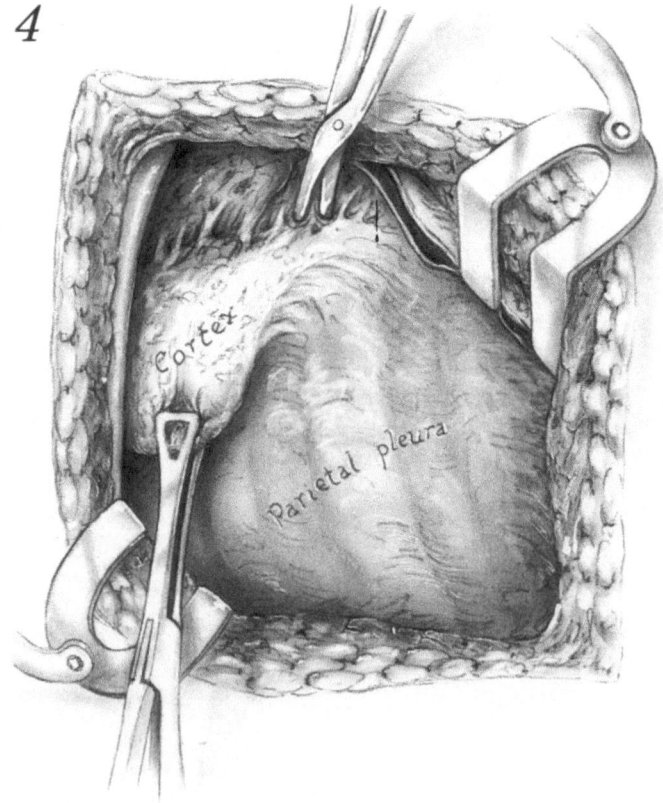

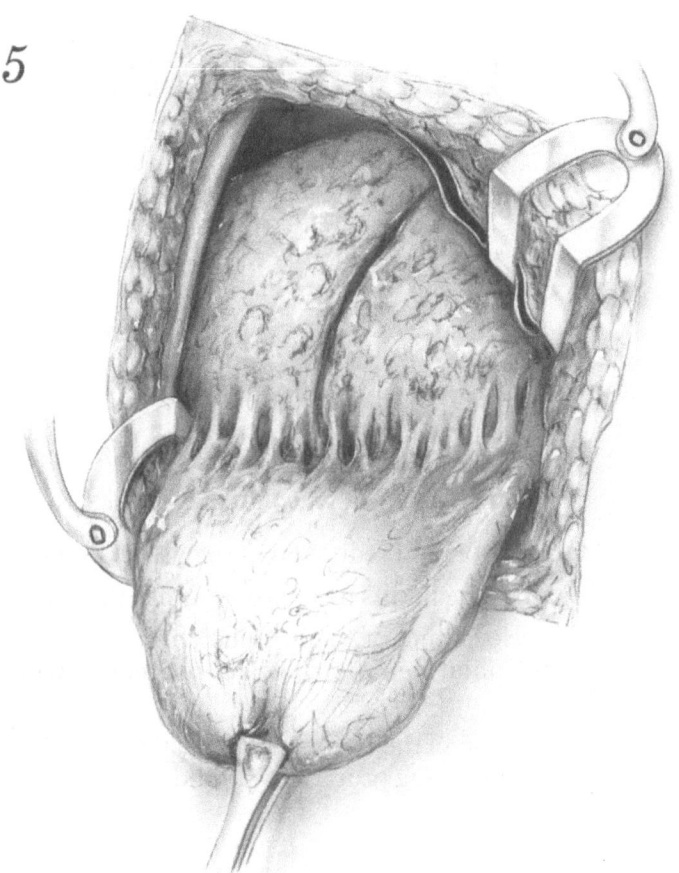

5 After virtual completion of the excision of the empyema, the underlying lung can be seen to expand to fill the hemithorax, and after complete removal of the empyema, the chest is closed routinely with drainage.

The incision is closed in layers with anterior and posterior drainage tubes with sideholes extending to the apex. The chest drains should not be clamped during transport of the patient back to the ward and care must be taken that the drains are not dislodged or kinked during movement. Once the patient is back in the ward the chest drains are connected to suction which must have careful control and be capable of high volume suction. Suction should be sufficient to maintain a negative pressure resulting in continuous bubbling throughout the respiratory cycle. Tubes are removed sequentially when all drainage and air leak has stopped.

Prophylactic antibiotics should be discontinued after 24 h. Antibiotics are thereafter only indicated for specific infective problems.

Adequate pain relief should be ensured to permit early and full movement of the shoulder and to allow the patient to co-operate with the physiotherapist in expectoration. Sputum problems are common following decortication, and if not dealt with promptly, will lead to life-threatening complications such as pulmonary infection. If sputum retention occurs despite adequate analgesia and intensive physiotherapy, suction bronchoscopy may be necessary. The insertion of a minitracheostomy tube through the cricothyroid membrane has largely replaced the performance of formal tracheostomy.

Cardiac dysrhythmias, particularly atrial tachycardias, are common following decortication and prophylactic digoxin is often used in the elderly.

With the emphasis on early mobilisation, deep venous thrombosis and pulmonary embolism are now rarities, and there is no evidence that low dose heparin is of any value.

15 Hiatus Hernia

Surgical control of pathological reflux entails:

1. Mobilisation and reduction of the associated hiatus hernia.
2. Repair of the hiatus by approximating the crura.
3. The performance of an anti-reflux procedure to buttress the weak lower oesophageal sphincter. For this final step the choice of procedure will vary. However, the initial steps are common to all.
4. If reduction of the hernia cannot be accomplished without tension on the repair, an oesophageal lengthening procedure should be interposed between steps 2 and 3.

Mobilisation and Reduction of the Hiatus Hernia

1

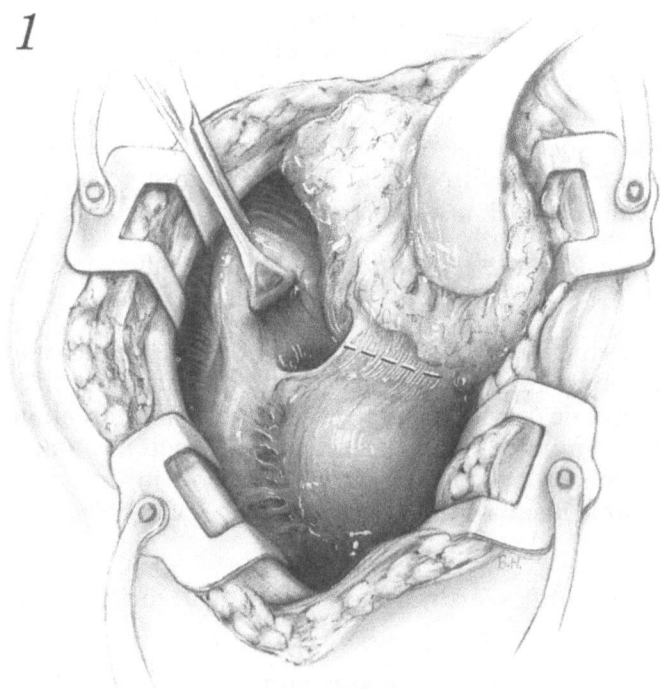

1 Access is via a left thoracotomy through the bed of the sixth rib. A double-lumen tube positioned in the left main bronchus allows collapse of the left lung, facilitating exposure. The hiatus hernia is seen as a fatty bulge at the hiatus beneath the mediastinal pleura. The lung is mobilised by division of the inferior pulmonary ligament.

2

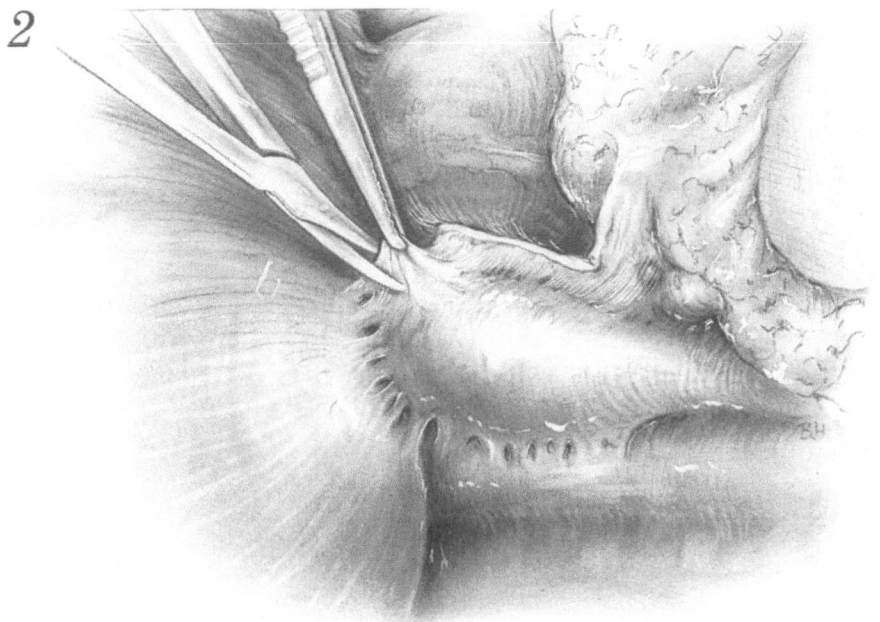

2 The mediastinal pleura is incised at the margin of the crura and dissection proceeds along the lateral aspect of the oesophagus to the inferior pulmonary vein. A tape passed around the oesophagus, encircling both vagus nerves, will aid later dissection.

3

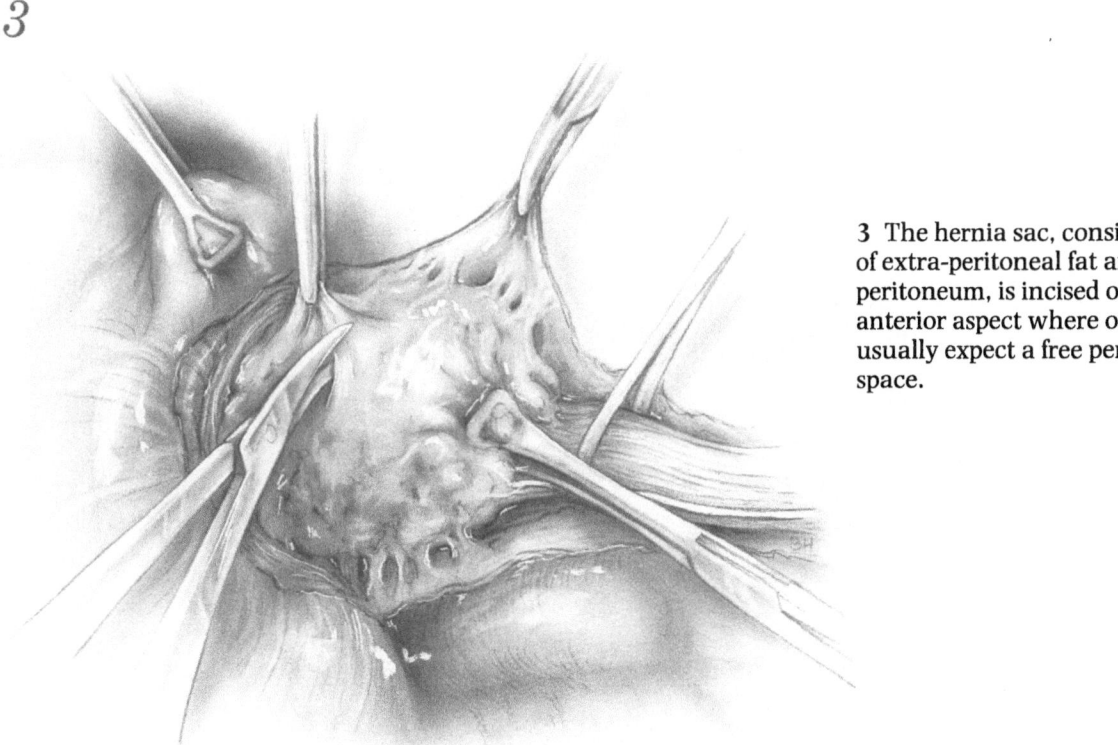

3 The hernia sac, consisting of extra-peritoneal fat and peritoneum, is incised on its anterior aspect where one can usually expect a free peritoneal space.

4

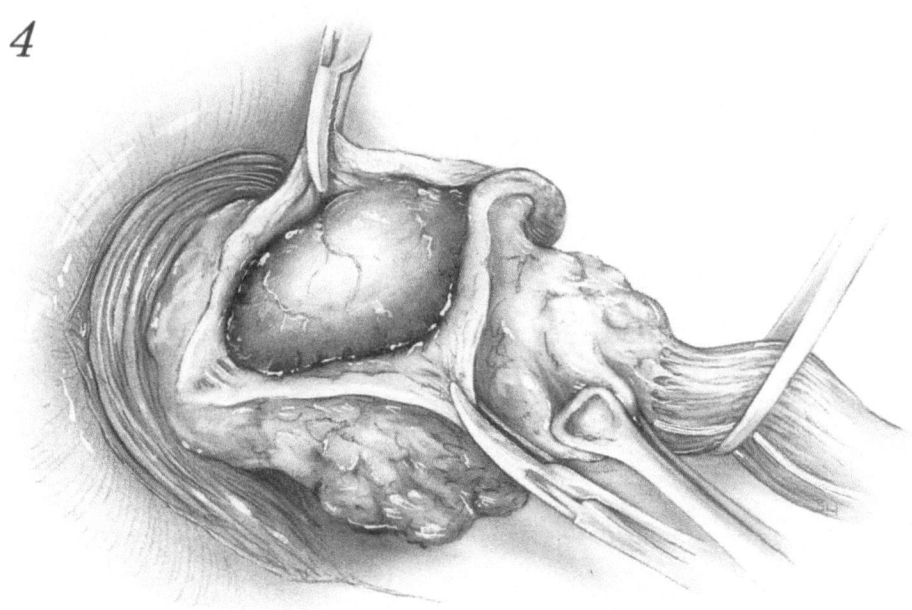

4, 5 Dissection continues around the hiatal margins, dividing the hiatal sac on to the posterior aspect of the stomach. Care needs to be taken not to damage the posterior vagus nerve as it fans out across the bare area of the stomach.

5

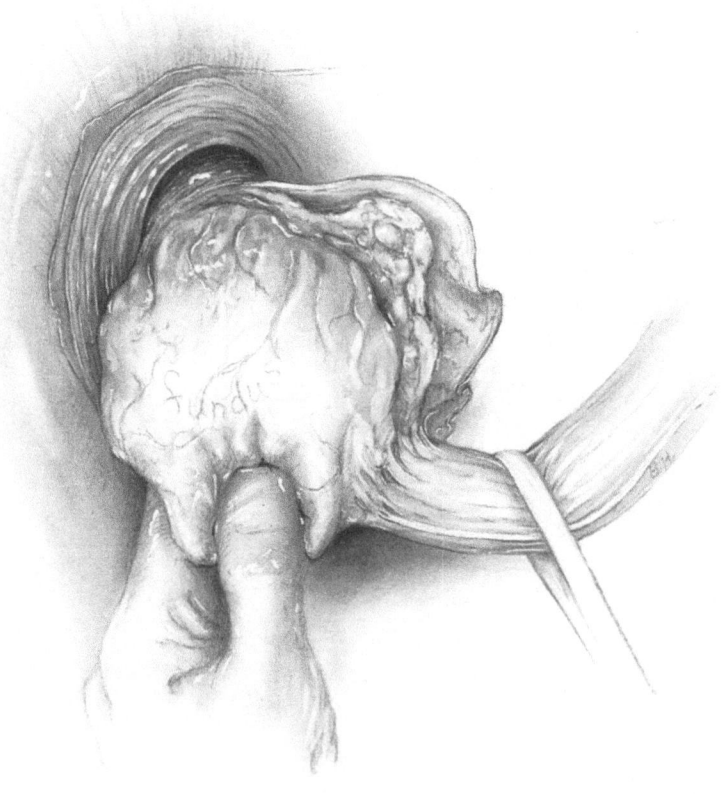

6

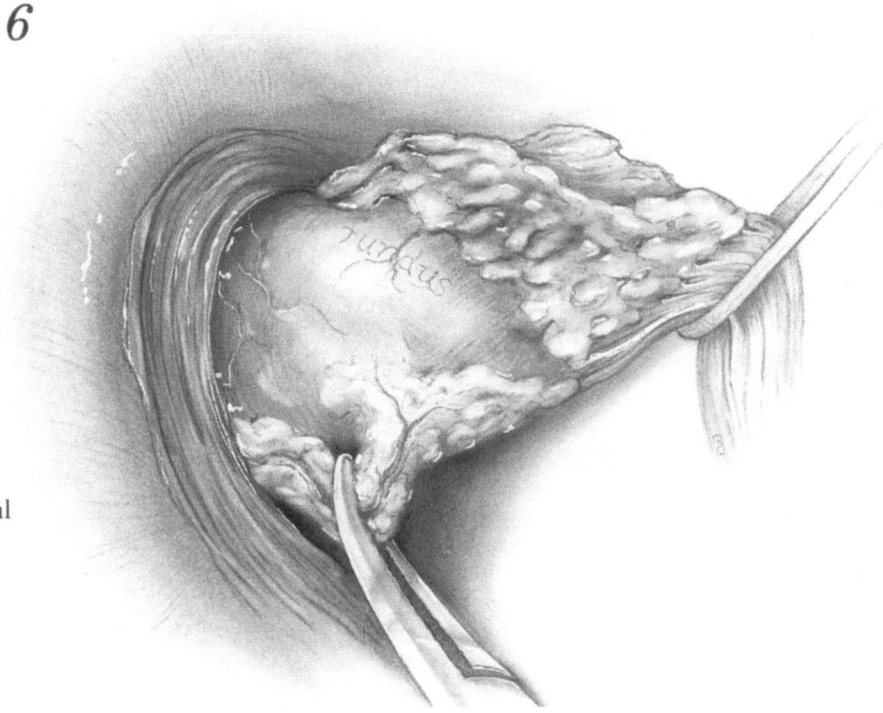

6 Whilst clearing the hiatal sac posteriorly over the bare area, the ascending branch of the left gastric artery will be encountered and it should be divided to free the fundus completely.

7

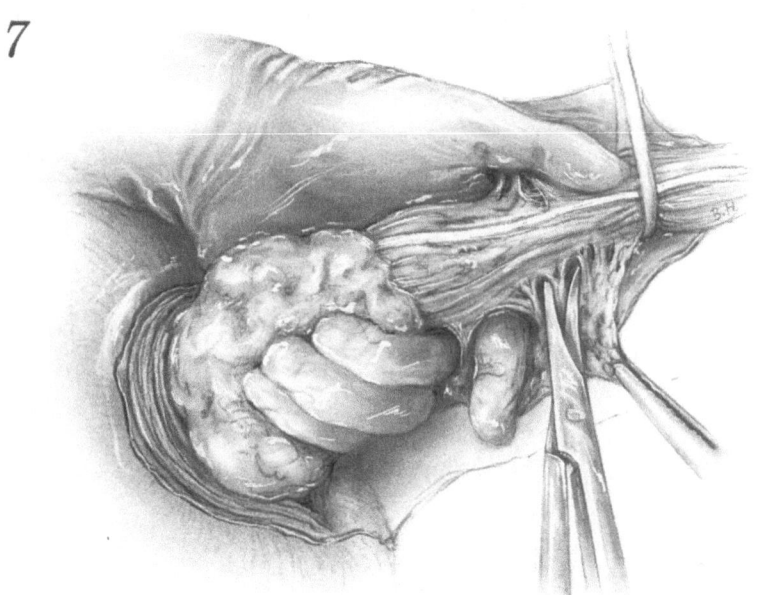

7 The stomach now freely moves through the hiatus. With traction on the tape the oesophagus is mobilised and the oesophageal branches of the aorta identified. If there is pan-mural oesophagitis this can be a difficult dissection. A sufficient length of the oesophagus should be mobilised to allow reduction of the stomach and repair without tension. One or more of the oesophageal branches of the aorta may be divided if necessary to permit reduction without tension. [If this procedure does not permit reduction without tension then an oesophageal lengthening procedure is recommended (Collis gastroplasty).]

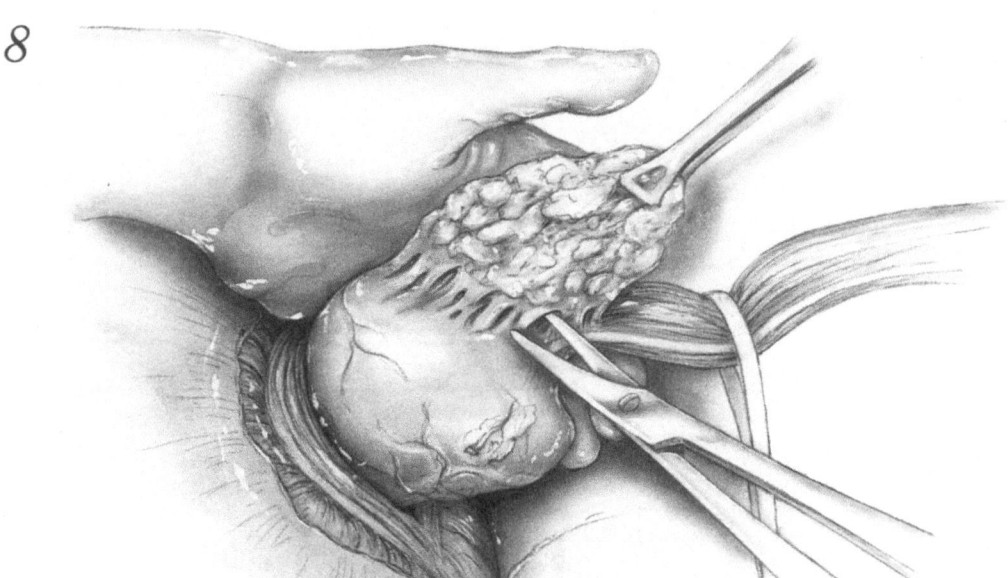

8 Extra-peritoneal fat and the hiatal sac are dissected from the lower oesophagus and proximal stomach to display clearly the position of the cardia. During this dissection special attention must be paid to the position of the vagus nerves so as not to damage them.

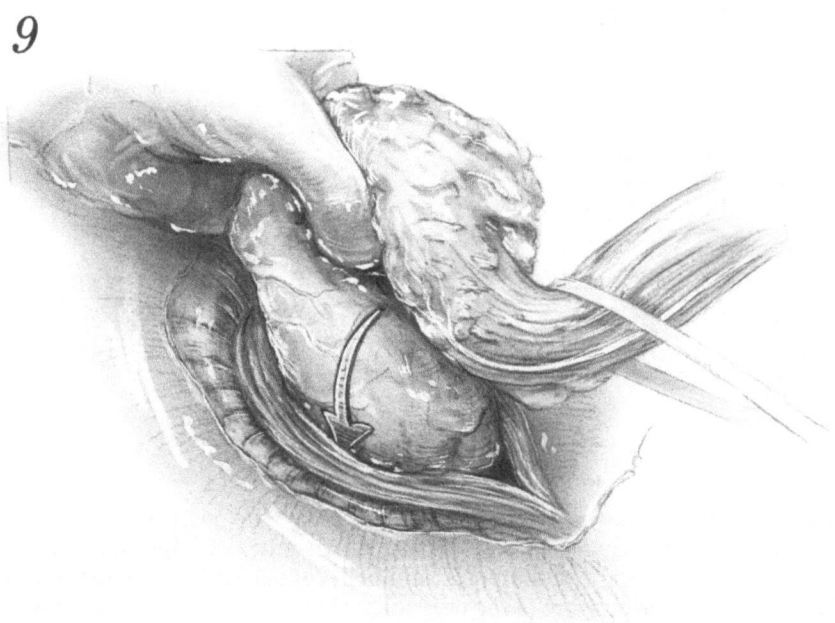

9 The stomach and cardia are then reduced into the abdomen without tension.

Repair of the Hiatus

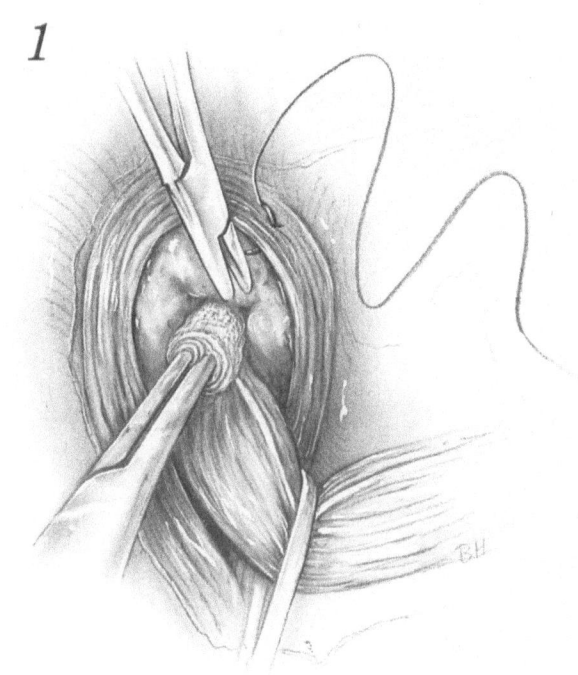

1

1 Braided non-absorbable sutures are used to approximate the crura. Good deep bites of the muscle should be taken. A mounted swab depresses the stomach, keeping it out of harm's way.

2

2 A single suture is used to approximate the crura anterior to the oesophagus and three or four posteriorly. *The sutures are not tied until the anti-reflux procedure has been performed.* (The surgeon should omit the crural suture anteriorly if a Belsey repair is intended.)

3

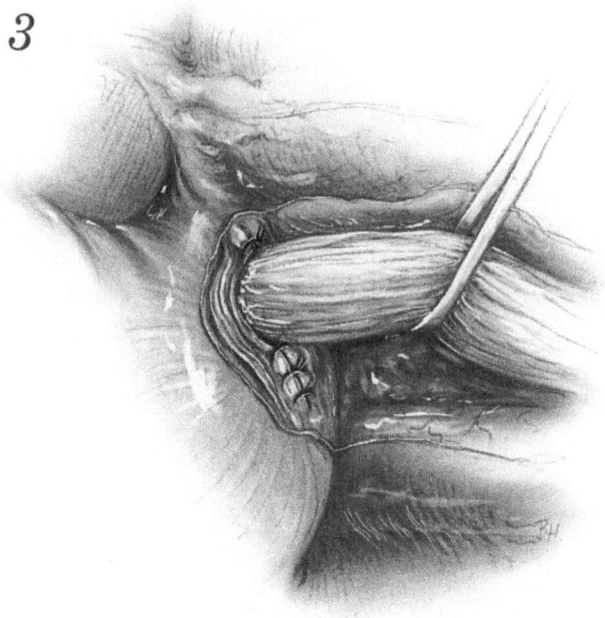

3 When the repair has been completed the stomach and repair are reduced into the abdomen. A large bougie (54 Fg Maloney) is then inserted into the oesophagus and the crural sutures are tied. The crura should be narrowed firmly but not tightly around the oesophagus containing the bougie. Having completed this step the bougie should be withdrawn and the hiatus should just admit the tip of the finger alongside the oesophagus.

Anti-reflux Procedures

Many techniques have been described which reinforce the hiatus hernia reduction and repair, helping control reflux and reducing the possibility of recurrence. The two illustrated here will serve in all circumstances. The Nissen fundoplication is simpler to understand and probably therefore more reliable. It may prove obstructive where oesophageal motility is impaired, e.g. achalasia or scleroderma, and in these circumstances the 270° wrap described by Belsey is preferred.

Nissen Fundoplication

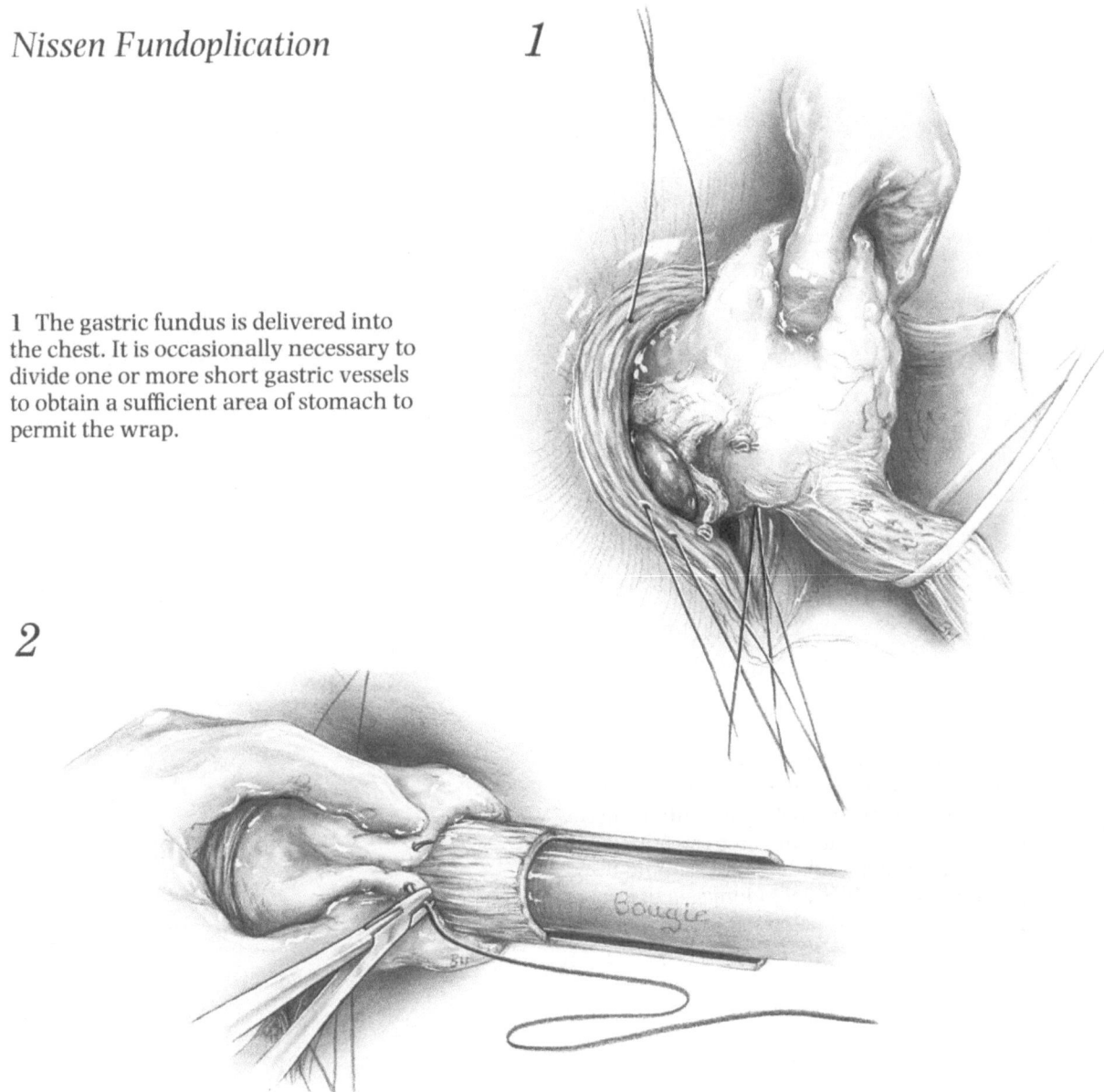

1 The gastric fundus is delivered into the chest. It is occasionally necessary to divide one or more short gastric vessels to obtain a sufficient area of stomach to permit the wrap.

2 A large bougie (54 Fg Maloney) is inserted into the oesophagus. The gastric fundus is wrapped around the cardia and lower oesophagus over an area of 2 3 cm. Stomach is sutured to stomach with non-absorbable braided suture to complete a 360° wrap. The most proximal suture should go through stomach, oesophageal muscle and stomach so as to prevent the wrap sliding down onto the stomach.

3

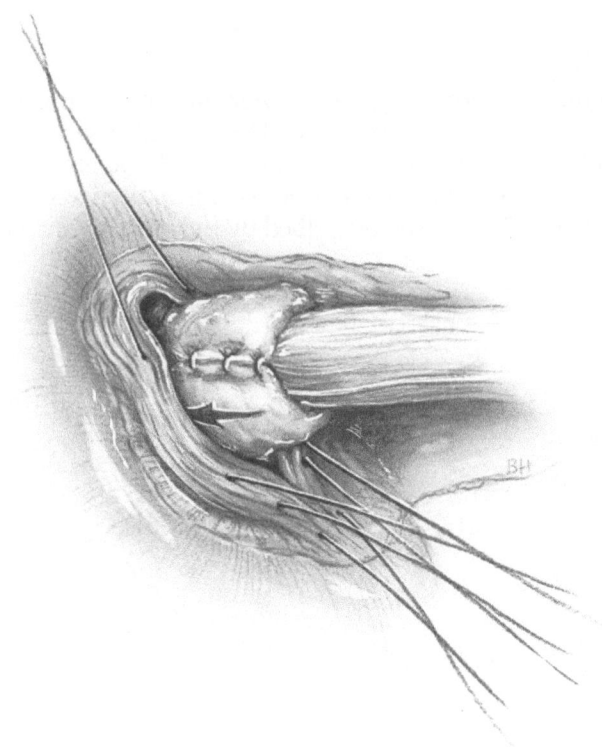

3 The completed repair is reduced into the abdomen without tension.

4

4 The previously placed crural sutures are now tied. The crura should be approximated firmly but not tightly around the oesophagus containing the bougie. Having completed this step the bougie should be withdrawn and the hiatus should now just admit the tip of the finger alongside the oesophagus.

Belsey Procedure

1

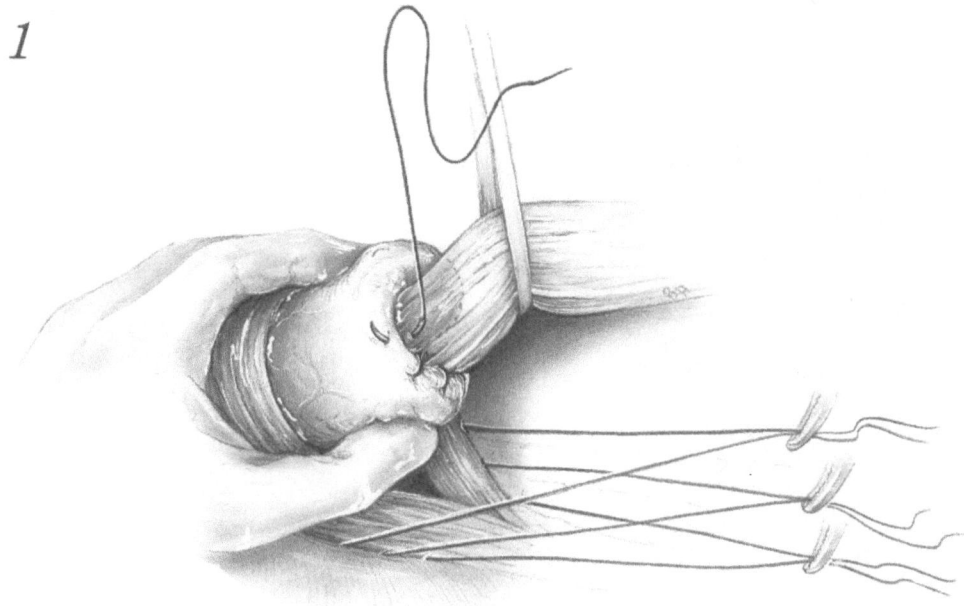

1 For this repair the crural sutures are all inserted posterior to the oesophagus. The stomach is rolled up onto the cardia and lower oesophagus on its anterior and lateral aspects to complete a 270° wrap. Two rows of interrupted non-absorbable braided sutures are used. The first row approximates stomach to oesophagus 1 cm above the cardia.

2

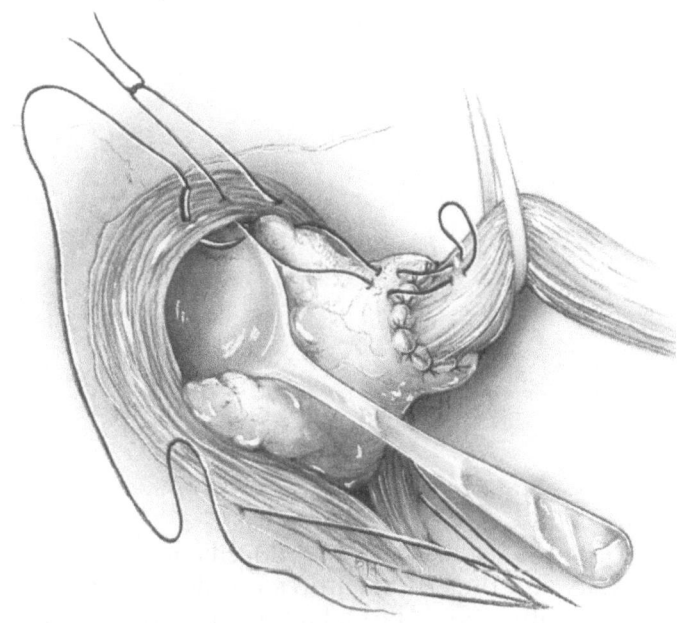

2 The second row of sutures is designed to roll the stomach a further 1 cm onto the anterior and lateral aspects of the lower oesophagus, but also incorporates diaphragm so as to fix the repair to the under-surface of the crura. Each suture passes through the crus, the stomach and the oesophagus and then loops to return through all three structures. All the sutures should be placed before any is tied.

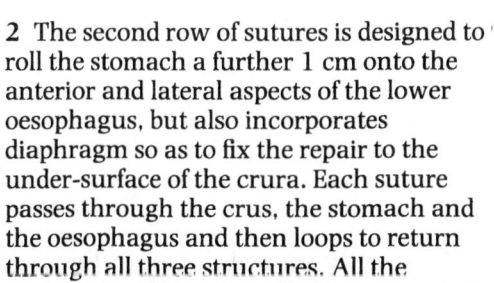

3

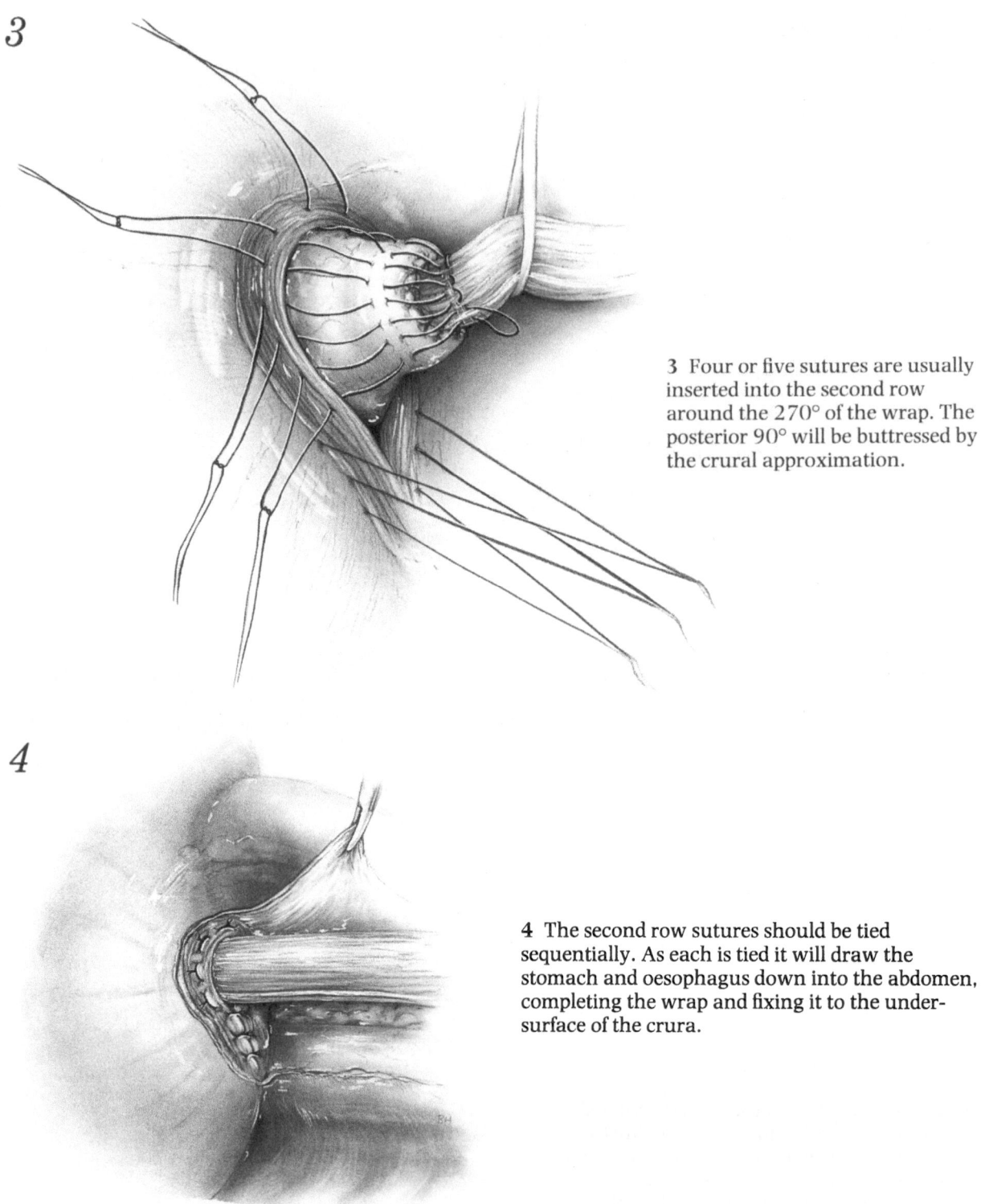

3 Four or five sutures are usually inserted into the second row around the 270° of the wrap. The posterior 90° will be buttressed by the crural approximation.

4

4 The second row sutures should be tied sequentially. As each is tied it will draw the stomach and oesophagus down into the abdomen, completing the wrap and fixing it to the under-surface of the crura.

Once the repair has been reduced a large bougie (54 Fg Maloney) is passed through the oesophagus and the crural sutures are tied firmly but not tightly around it. On removing the bougie the hiatus should just admit the tip of the finger posteriorly alongside the oesophagus.

Lengthening the Oesophagus by Collis Gastroplasty (Optional)

The Collis gastroplasty effectively lengthens the oesophagus by producing a gastric tube. Where oesophagitis has caused shortening of the oesophagus it allows reduction of the repair without undue tension. This manoeuvre is undertaken following insertion of the crural sutures, but prior to performing the anti-reflux procedure.

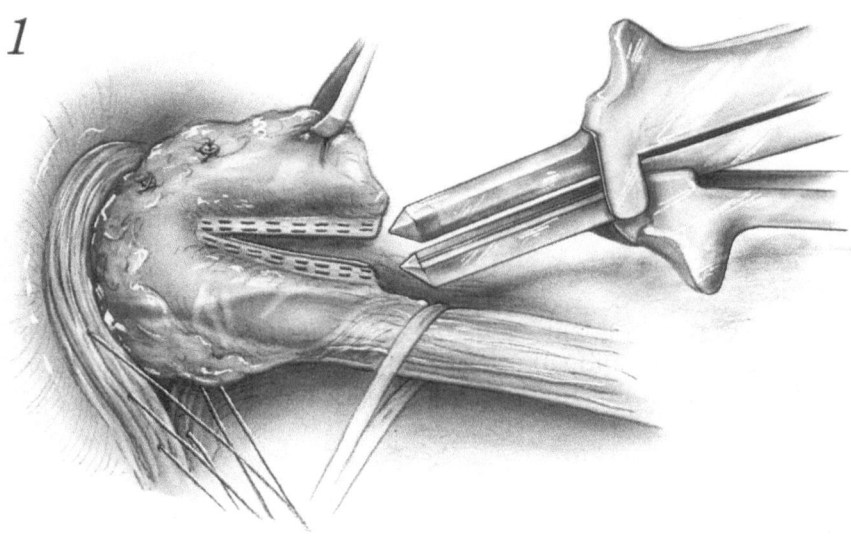

1

1 A large bougie (60 Fg Maloney) is inserted into the oesophagus. A gastric tube is fashioned by incising into the stomach from the angle between the fundus and the cardia for a distance of 2–3 cm. This may be performed using clamps, but is facilitated by a linear stapler which also cuts between the rows of staples.

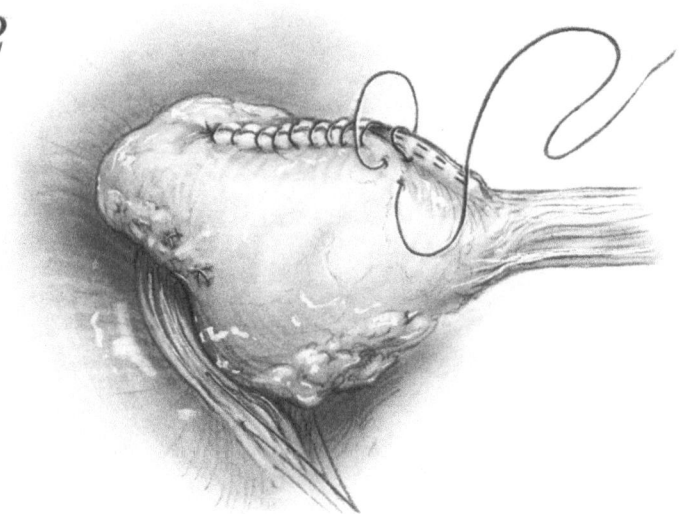

2

2 The row of staples is oversewn using a continuous suture of non-absorbable braided material. The V-incision thus becomes a linear repair.

3

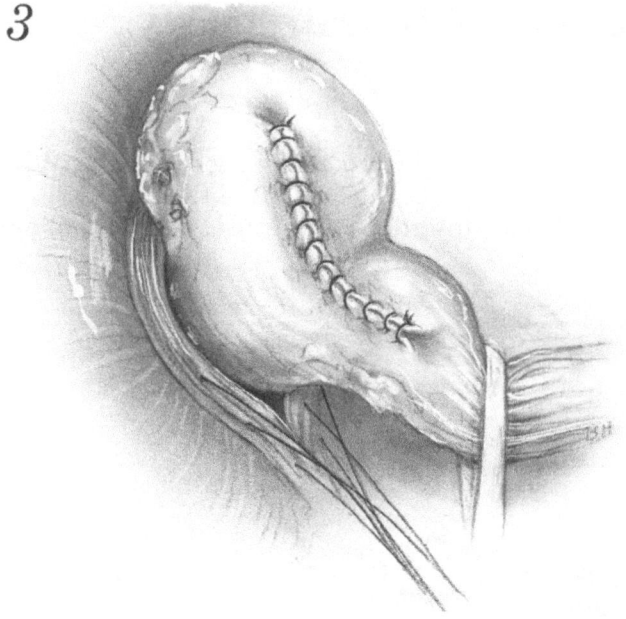

3 The Collis gastroplasty may be an additional step prior to a Nissen fundoplication. The incised fundus permits fundoplication without difficulty, the wrap being performed around the gastric tube and lower cardia.

There is no need for a nasogastric tube following this operation unless the surgeon fears he may have damaged the vagus nerves. Swallowing may commence on the first post-operative day. Some dysphagia for solids may occur during the first 2 weeks. If it persists after this period, gentle bougienage may be necessary.

16 Colon Interposition

The place of this operation is yet to be defined. It is no longer popular for the relief of malignant obstruction of the oesophagus. It has been traditionally used to relieve benign but irreversible strictures of the oesophagus. A short segment colon interposition may be used to replace the lower oesophagus scarred and shortened by chronic reflux. It is becoming increasingly appreciated that many such "irreversible" strictures may recover with satisfactory surgical control of reflux, usually aided by oesophageal lengthening procedures. A long segment colon interposition may be used to replace the whole oesophagus and even the distal pharynx. Such extensive resection may prove necessary following caustic ingestion or for refractory motility problems. Even this role for colonic interposition is under attack from some who believe that better long-term swallowing may be achieved by the simpler and safer procedures carrying a gastric conduit to the neck. Despite this, colonic interposition remains a useful part of the surgical armamentarium and good long-term results have been reported.

The operation described below is that of short segment colonic interposition to replace a long benign stricture due to reflux and associated with considerable shortening of the oesophagus. Bowel preparation requires only that a low residue diet be given for 3 days prior to surgery. Antibiotic preparation of the colon is unnecessary. Prophylactic antibiotics are commenced with the premedication, using parenteral agents effective against the aerobic and anaerobic organisms found in the colon and obstructed oesophagus.

If there has been no previous abdominal surgery this operation may, with experience, be performed through a left thoracotomy. The inexperienced surgeon is recommended to undertake left thoraco-laparotomy.

An endobronchial tube passed by the anaesthetist will facilitate intrathoracic dissection by allowing collapse of the left lung.

1

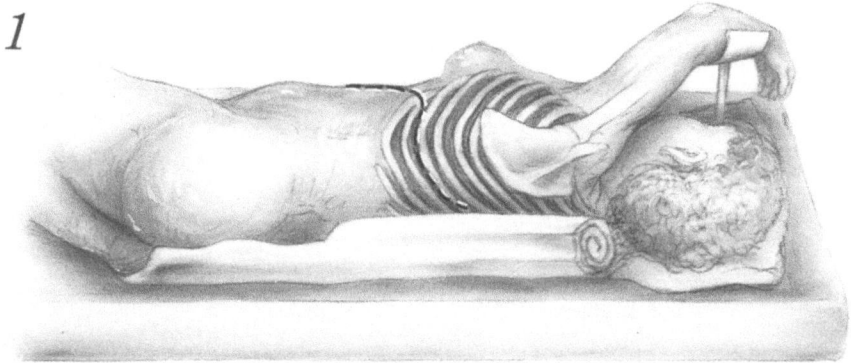

1 The patient is positioned in the left anterior oblique position with a support beneath the spine. The scapula is rotated from the operative field by supporting the arm on a rest above the head. A long oblique incision is made from the linea alba, midway between xiphoid and umbilicus, diagonally to the costal margin and along the line of the eighth rib beneath the tip of the scapula.

2

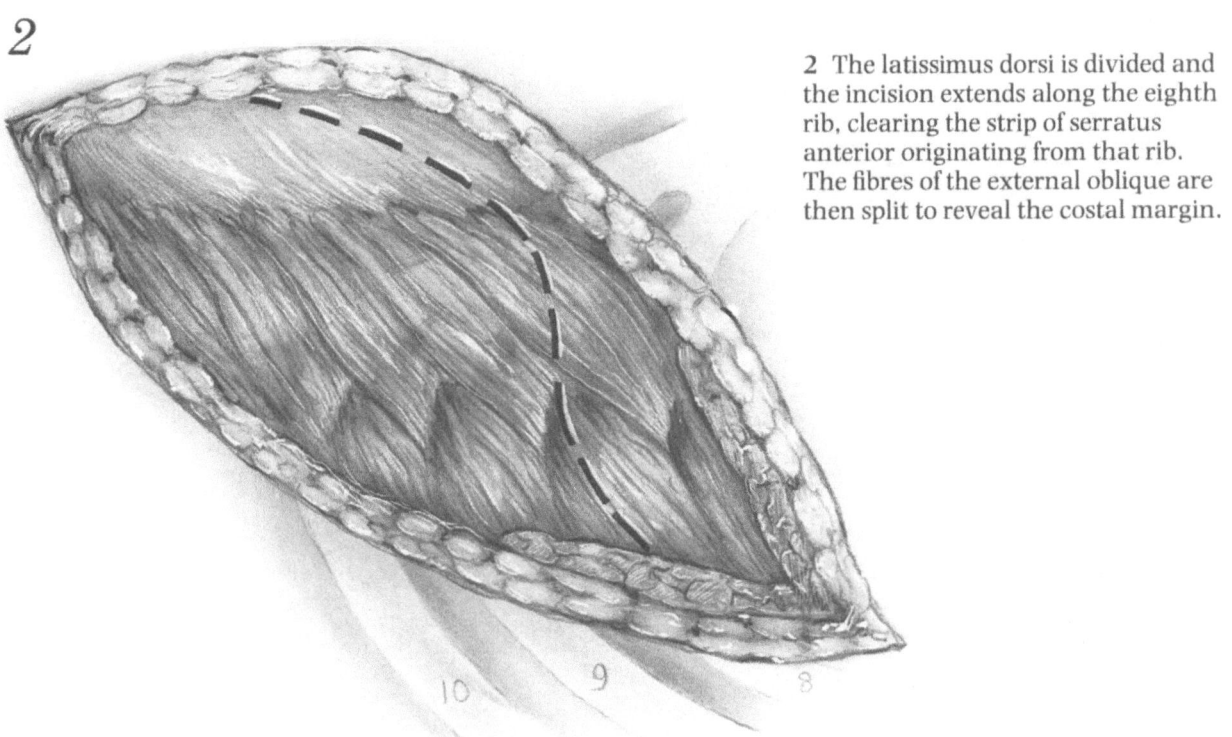

2 The latissimus dorsi is divided and the incision extends along the eighth rib, clearing the strip of serratus anterior originating from that rib. The fibres of the external oblique are then split to reveal the costal margin.

3

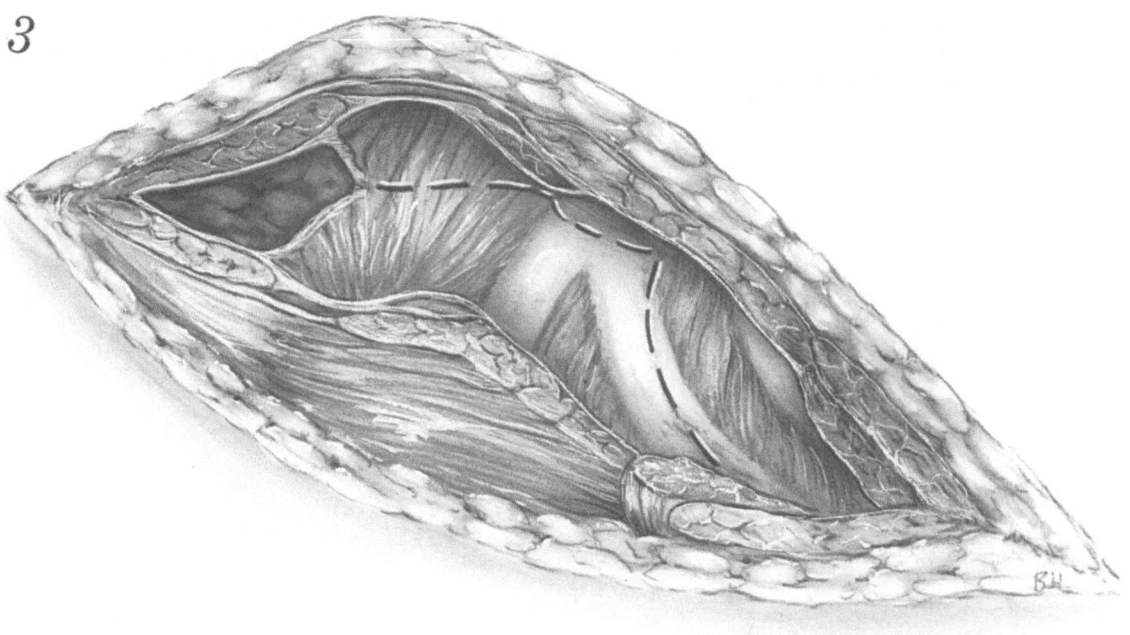

3 The abdominal muscles are divided and the costal cartilage divided using the diathermy. The superior epigastric artery and the costo-diaphragmatic vessels require control. The pleural and peritoneal spaces are opened in the line of the incision. The diaphragm is divided beneath the costal margin, passing circumferentially to skirt the central tendon.

4

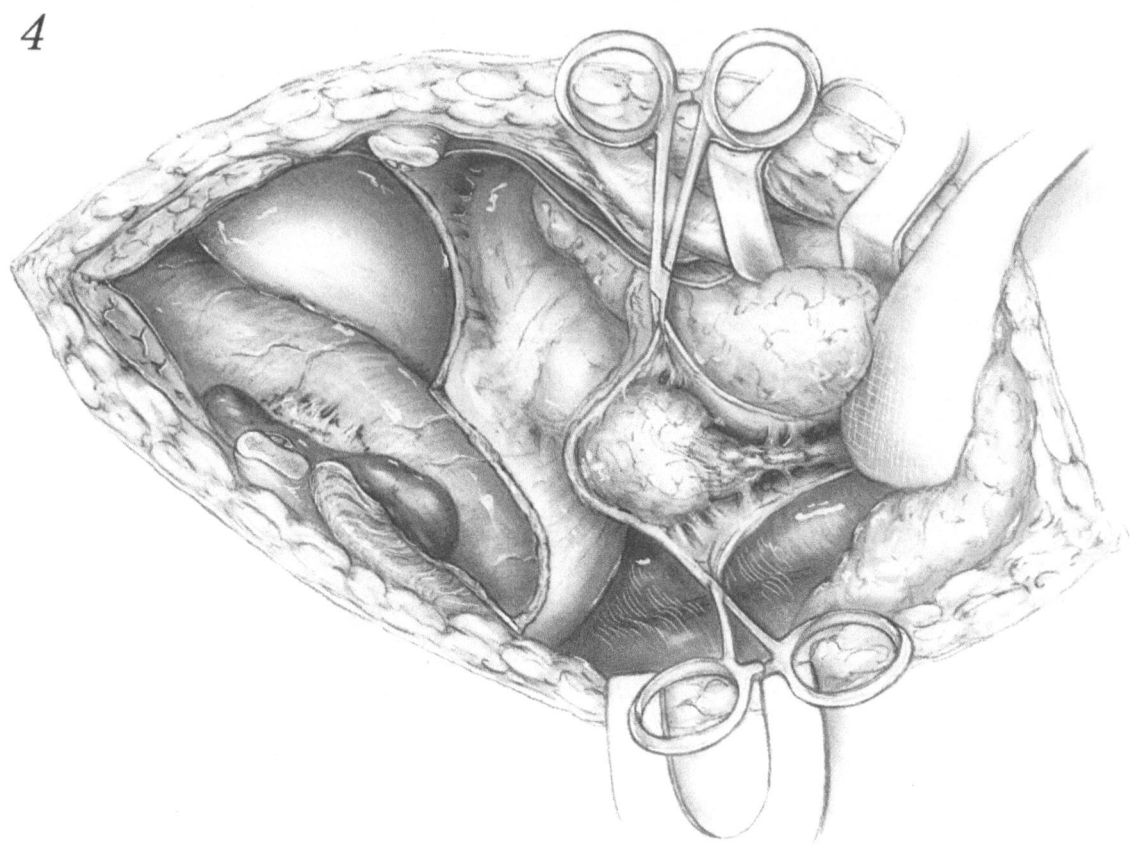

4 The parietal pleura is opened over the oesophagus. The diseased segment of oesophagus is mobilised superiorly until normal oesophagus is encountered. Dissection then proceeds inferiorly to the oesophageal hiatus. Both vagus nerves are divided.

5

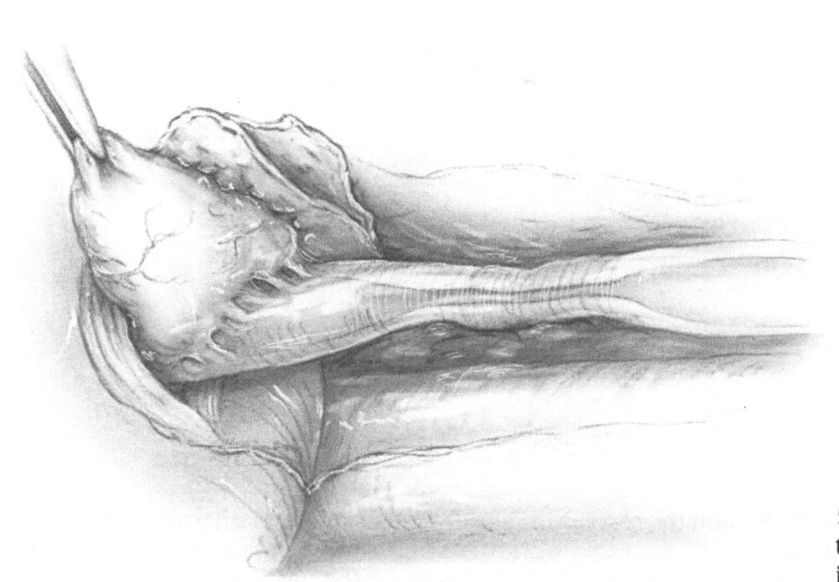

5 The hernia sac is opened and the gastro-oesophageal junction is defined.

6

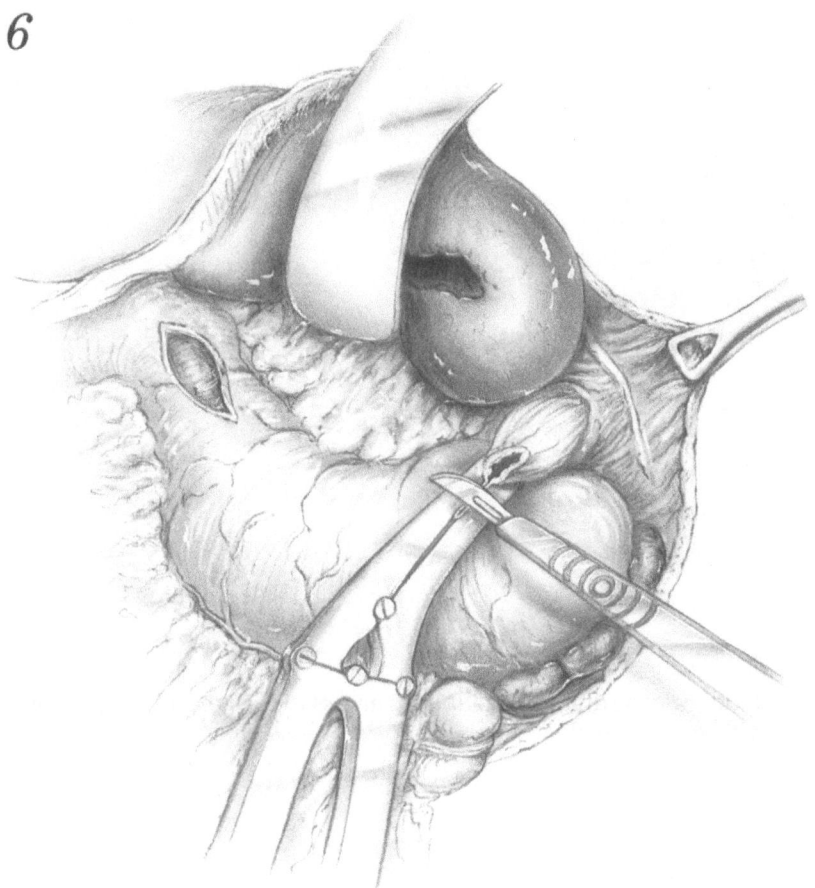

6 A Peyr's clamp is applied on the gastric side of the cardia and the cardia transected. A pyloroplasty, or pyloro-myotomy is performed.

7

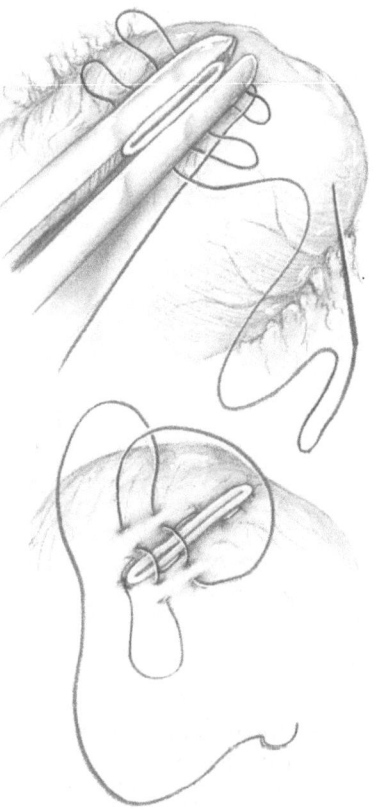

7 The stomach is closed using a sewing machine suture of absorbable material and the crushed flange is then inverted with a continuous over and over non-absorbable suture.

8

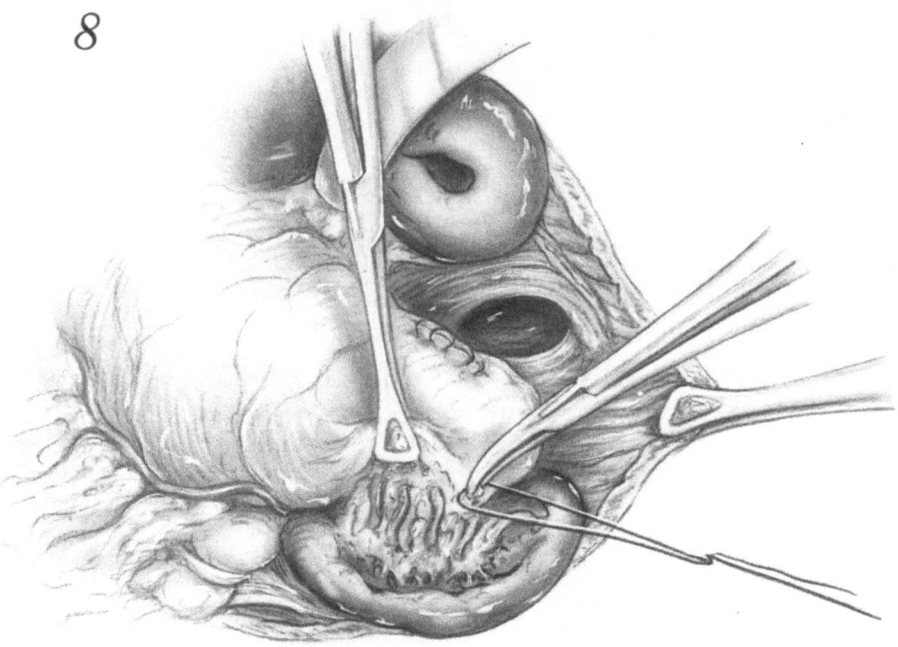

8 One or more of the short gastric arteries may be divided, facilitating access to the posterior aspect of the stomach where the anastomosis will be performed.

9

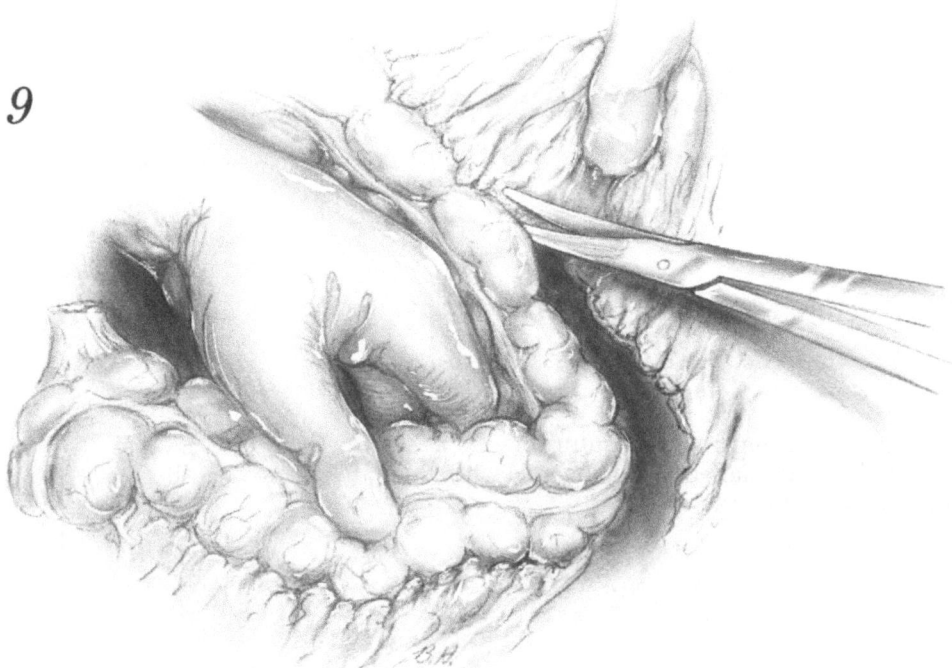

9 Mobilisation of the colon commences by detaching the greater omentum from the superior margin of the transverse colon. There should be little bleeding. The splenic flexure and descending colon may be mobilised by division of the peritoneal reflection.

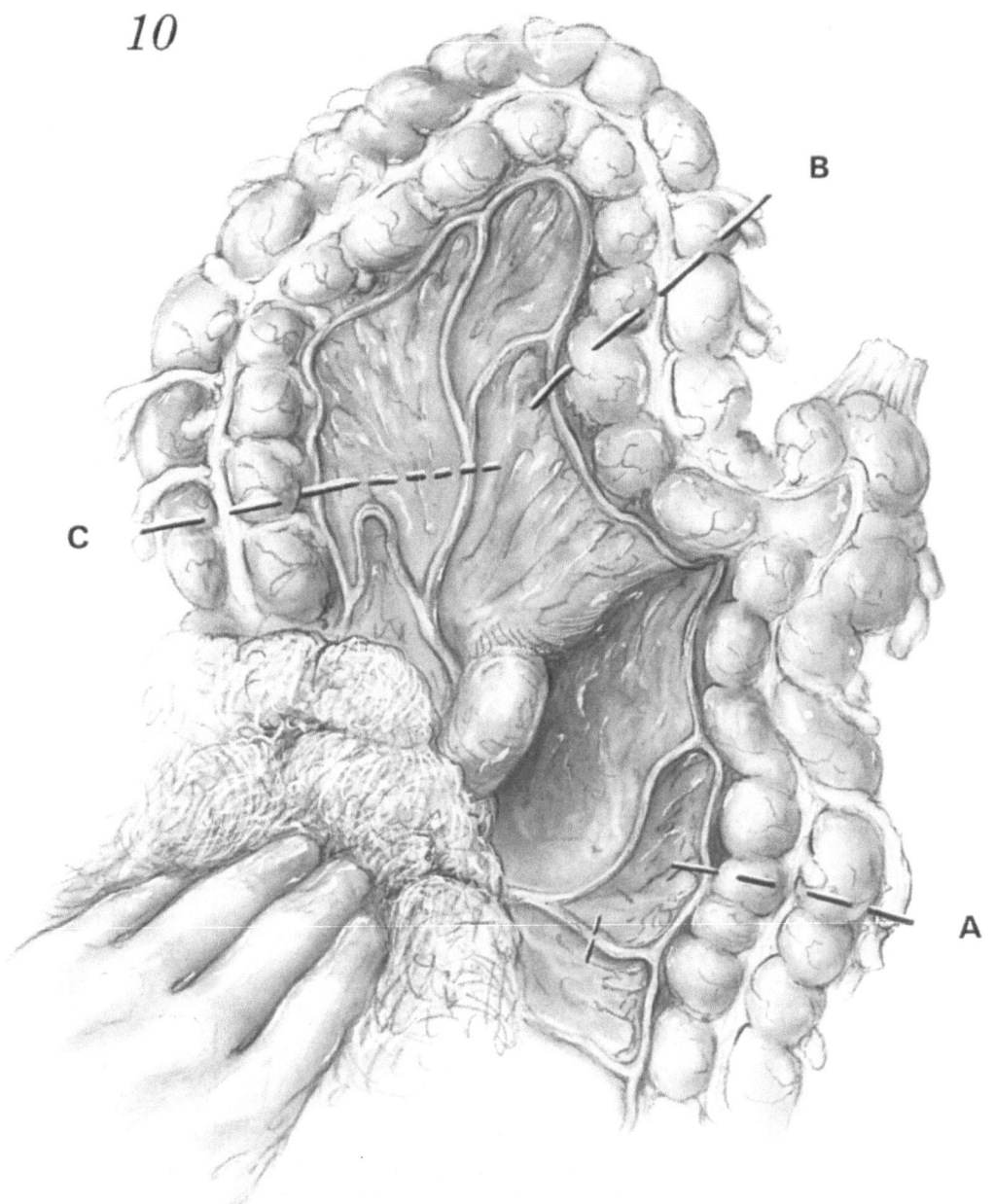

10 The vascular supply of the colon should then be carefully studied so as to achieve the desired length, preserving the marginal artery. If the marginal vessels are incomplete another conduit should be chosen. For short segment colon interposition the left half of the transverse colon and the splenic flexure may be mobilised (A-B), preserving the ascending branch of the left colic artery. For longer segments the middle colic artery may be divided so as to use the whole length of the transverse colon (A-C).

11

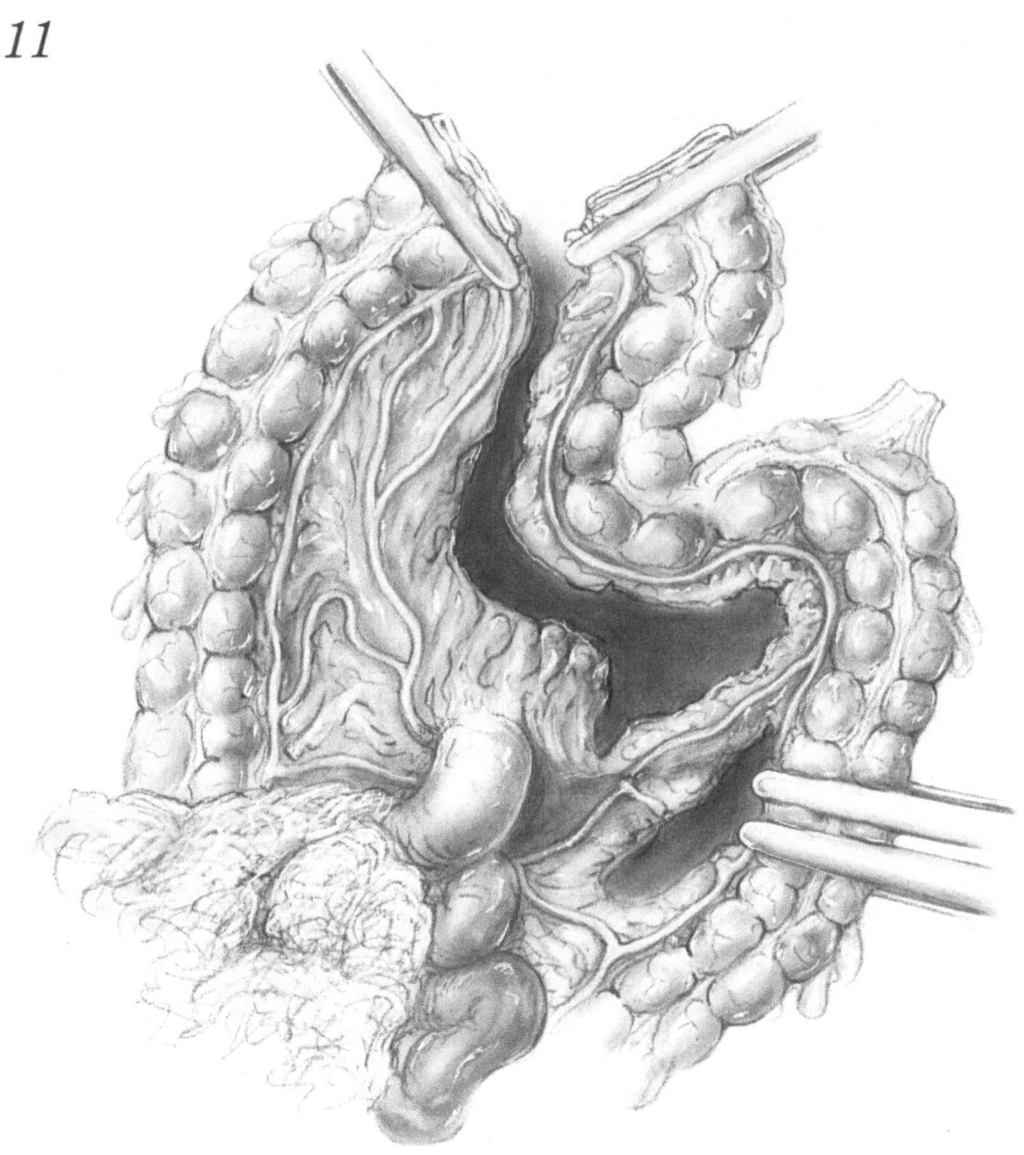

11 Once a suitable length of colon has been isolated the marginal artery may be divided. If this is undertaken without haemostats, brisk bleeding should occur from the isolated loop and this is reassuring. Any faecal material within the segment is milked distally. Soft occlusion clamps are applied at the lines of transection and the colon divided.

12

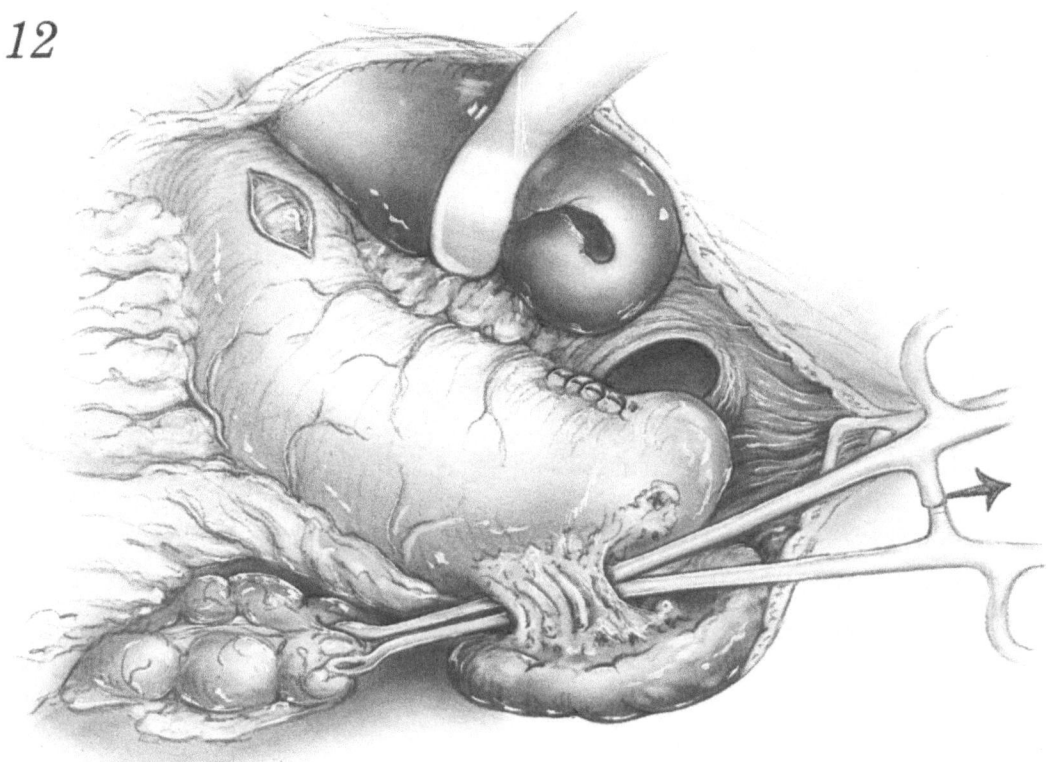

12 The proximal end of the colon is passed behind the stomach through the oesophageal hiatus so as to position the bowel in an isoperistaltic fashion. The hiatus may have to be enlarged to accommodate the colon.

13

13 The distal oesophagus may be spatulated to overcome any discrepancy with the diameter of the colon. An end to end oesophago-colic anastomosis is undertaken using a continuous suture of 3.0 monofilament non-absorbable material.

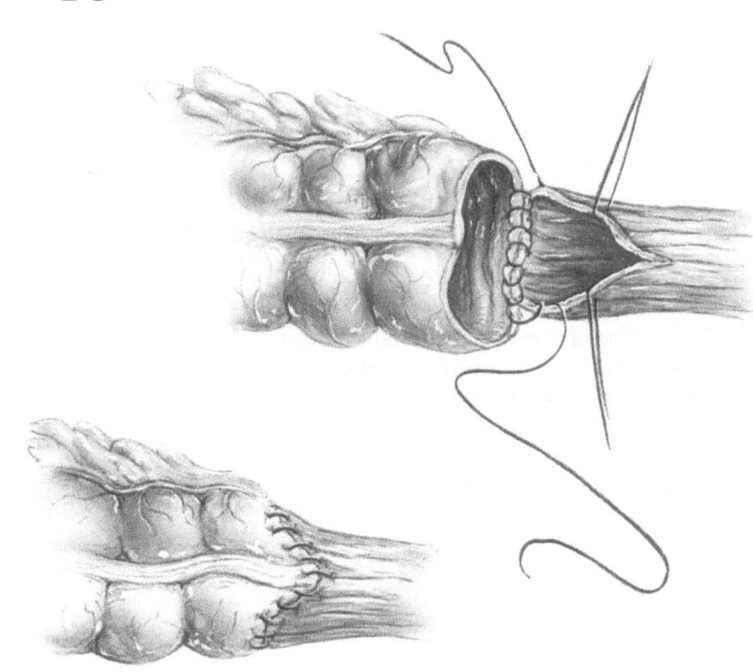

14

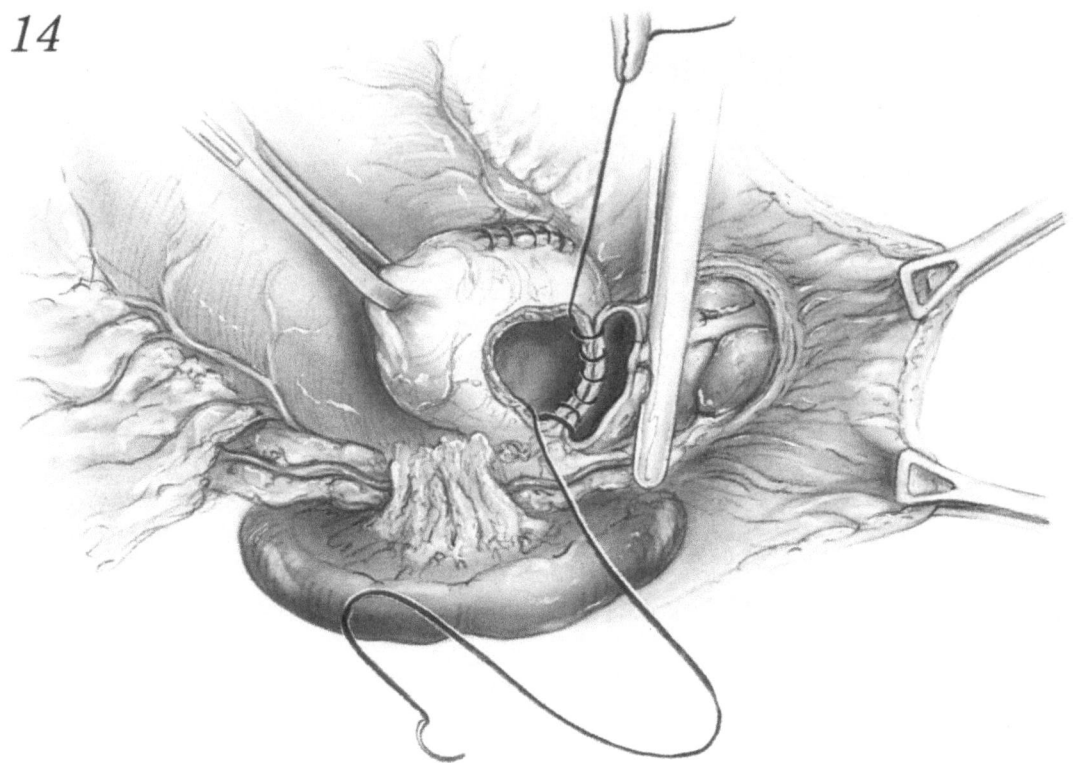

14 The stomach is reflected anteriorly and a suitable site for anastomosis is selected on the posterior wall, well away from the gastric closure. A disc of stomach is excised and the gastro-colic anastomosis performed with a continuous suture of 3.0 monofilament non-absorbable material. A nasogastric tube is passed by the anaesthetist, manipulated through the colonic segment by the surgeon and positioned in the stomach prior to completion of this anastomosis.

15

15 This anastomosis is then invaginated using interrupted non-absorbable sutures to draw the fundus onto the intra-abdominal portion of the colonic segment. This will reinforce the anastomosis and by maintaining an intra-abdominal segment of colon may have an anti-reflux function.

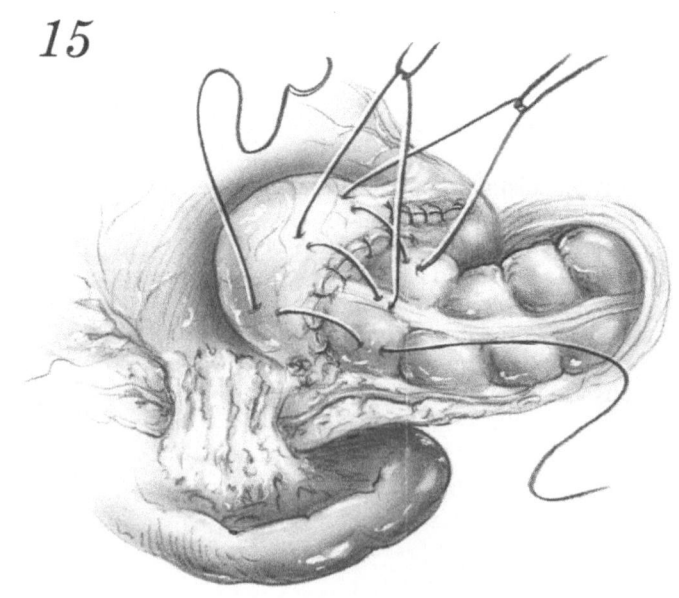

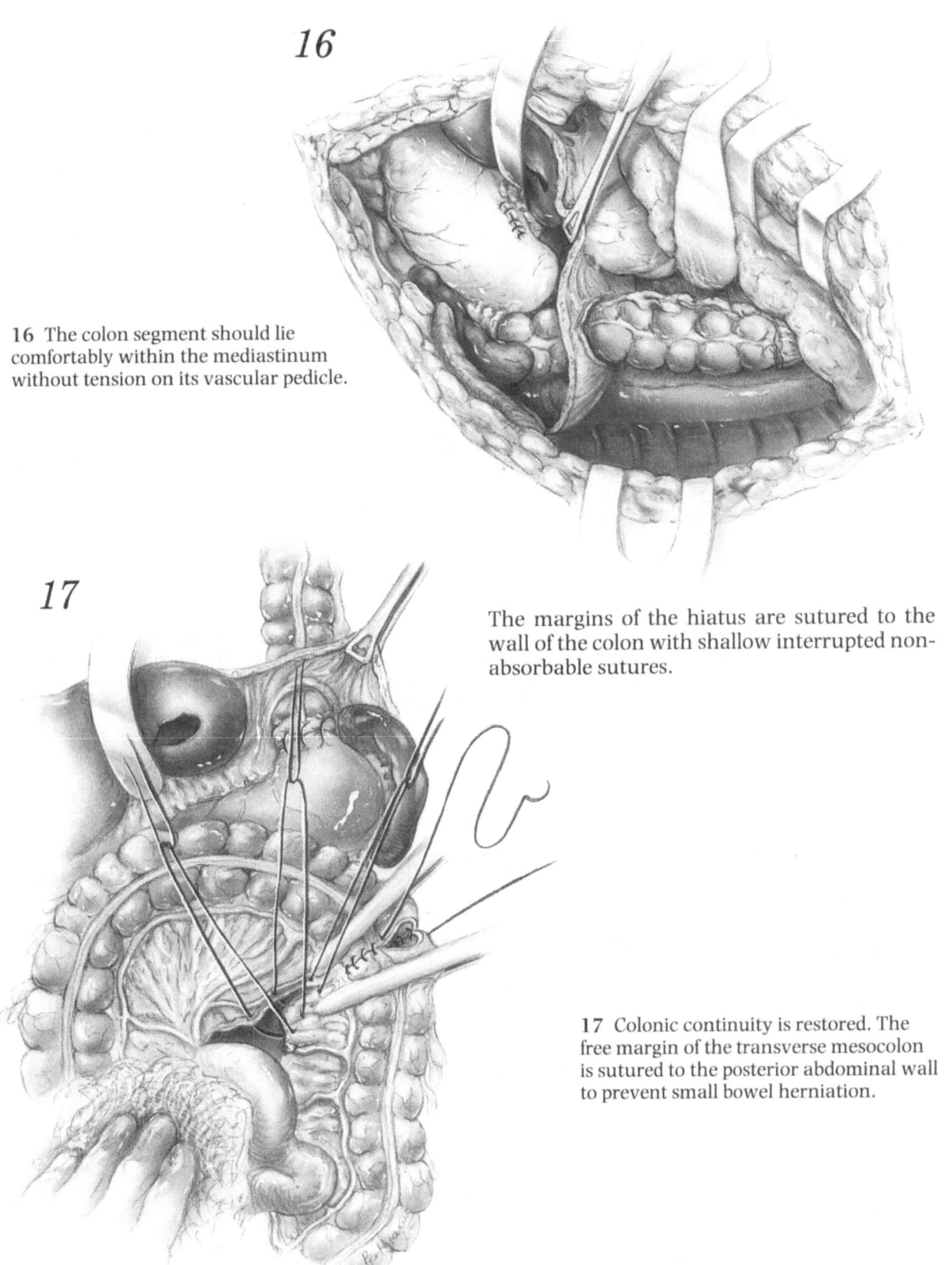

16 The colon segment should lie comfortably within the mediastinum without tension on its vascular pedicle.

The margins of the hiatus are sutured to the wall of the colon with shallow interrupted non-absorbable sutures.

17 Colonic continuity is restored. The free margin of the transverse mesocolon is sutured to the posterior abdominal wall to prevent small bowel herniation.

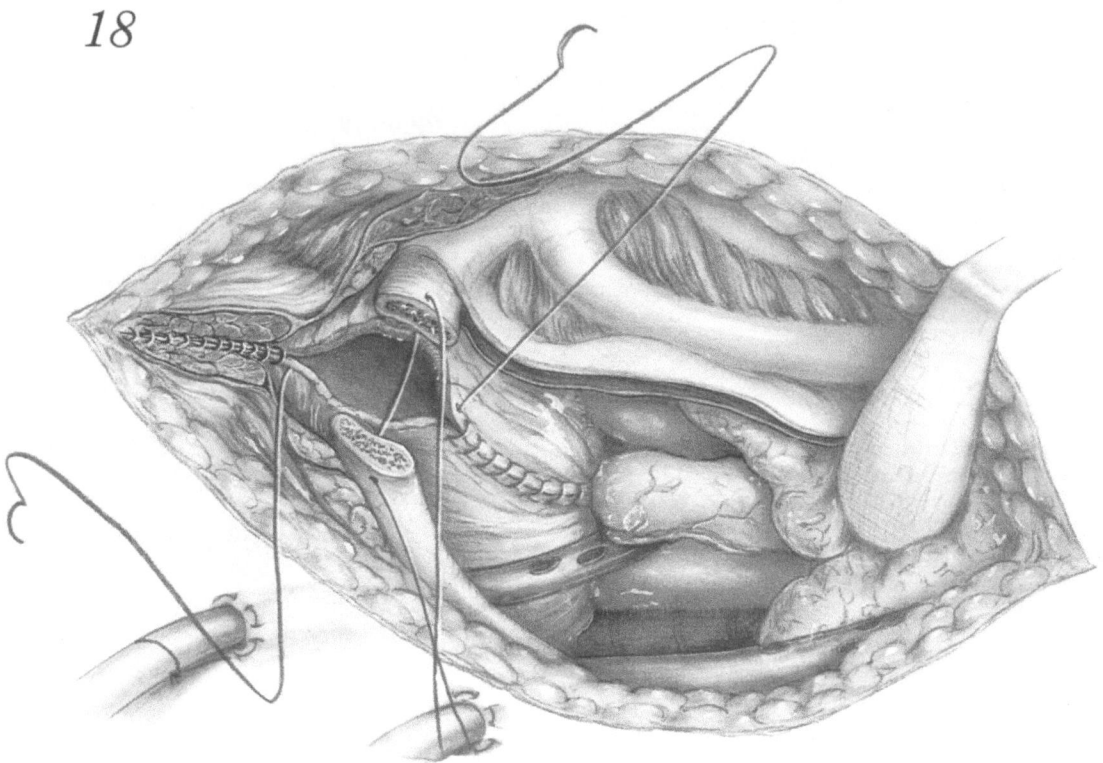

18 The thoracolaparotomy wound is now closed. Closure of the diaphragm continues on to the posterior oblique muscles. Two chest drains are required, one of which may pass across the mediastinum to drain the right pleural space if opened. The ribs and costal margin are approximated using interrupted sutures. The muscles of the chest and abdominal walls are then closed in layers.

The nasogastric tube may be removed once gastric emptying is assured, usually by the second post-operative day. Ileus is most unusual beyond this period and oral feeding may therefore be commenced.

Antibiotics are discontinued after 24 h unless a specific infective problem arises.

17 Achalasia

Longitudinal myotomy of the lower oesophagus and cardia (Heller's operation) provides good palliation for troublesome achalasia. It does not, of course, correct the underlying defect, merely vandalising the normal anti-reflux mechanisms. Combining this operation with an anti-reflux operation is somewhat illogical, merely going full circle. It can only be successful since our artificial anti-reflux procedures are less obstructive, and less competent, than the lower oesophageal sphincter.

The relative merits of myotomy versus hydrostatic bougienage are beyond the scope of this book. Many surgeons reserve myotomy for those patients inadequately or only temporarily helped by bougienage.

The timing of surgery is difficult since many sufferers are unaware of their swallowing abnormality. If dysphagia is severe and associated with weight loss then the position is clear. Often, however, the decision is based upon progressive dilatation of the oesophagus over a prolonged period of observation.

A similar, more extensive, myotomy may be undertaken for diffuse oesophageal spasm.

1

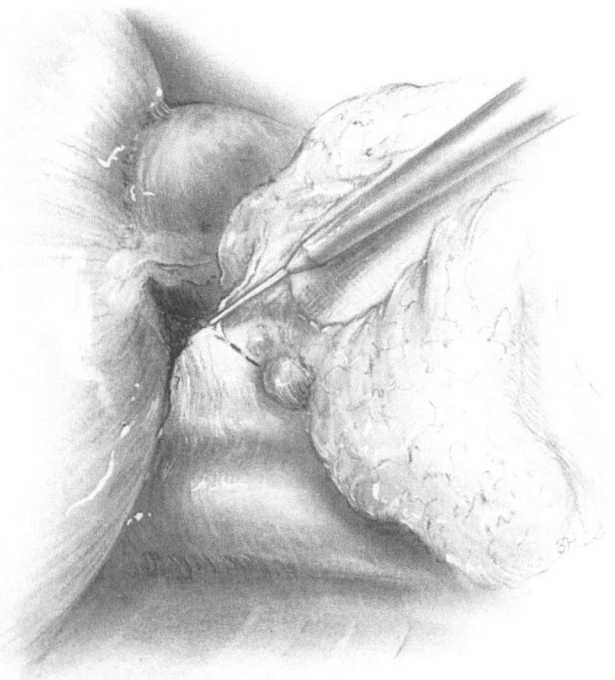

1 Access is via a left thoracotomy through the bed of the sixth rib. An endobronchial tube into the left main bronchus allows collapse of the left lung, facilitating exposure. The lung is mobilised by division of the inferior pulmonary ligament.

2

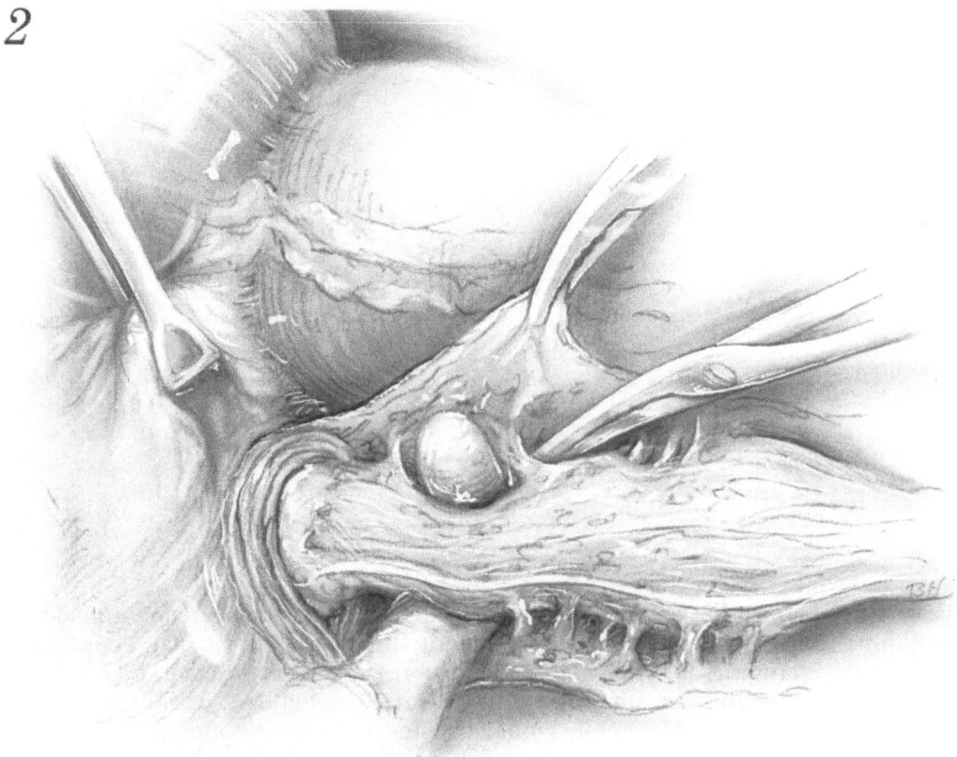

2 The mediastinal pleura is opened along the lateral aspects of the oesophagus. The grossly thickened and dilated oesophagus is mobilised with blunt and sharp dissection. Where there is mega-oesophagus this step may prove difficult. The vagus nerves are identified. A tape encircles the oesophagus, excluding the vagus nerves.

3

3 A longitudinal myotomy is undertaken, commencing on the lower oesophagus. Gentle strokes of the knife will divide the longitudinal muscle to disclose the underlying circular fibres. Traction on the tape will allow a few millimetres of the stomach to herniate into the chest without disrupting the hiatus permanently.

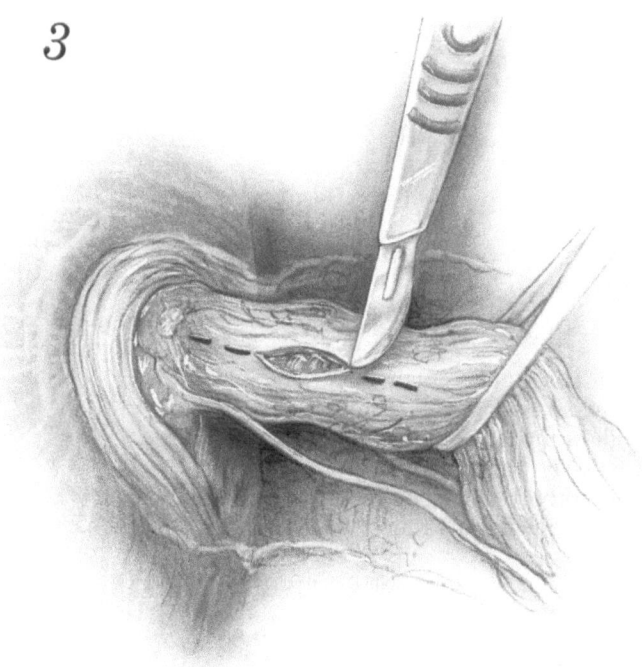

4

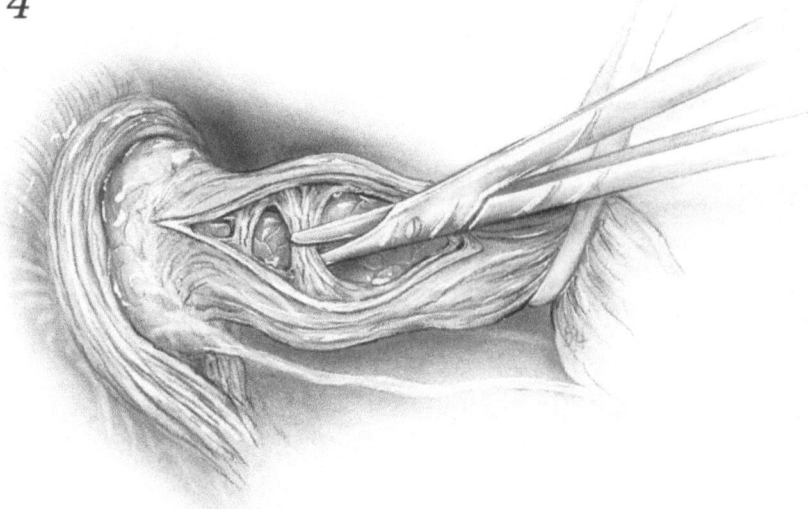

4 The submucosal vascular bed is clearly seen and any final strands of circular muscle can be divided with scissors. The myotomy is continued inferiorly for 2–3 mm onto the proximal stomach. The stomach can be usually identified by the change in direction of the muscle fibres. Great care must be taken at this point as the stomach wall is often thinner than that of the abnormal oesophagus and the mucosa may be damaged. The myotomy continues proximally for at least 5 cm onto the oesophagus. If there is diffuse oesophageal spasm, the myotomy must be performed along the length of oesophagus where motility has been shown to be abnormal on manometry.

5

5 The margins of the myotomy are swept laterally using blunt dissection, allowing the mucosal tube to herniate through the myotomy. A careful search should be made for any mucosal defects.

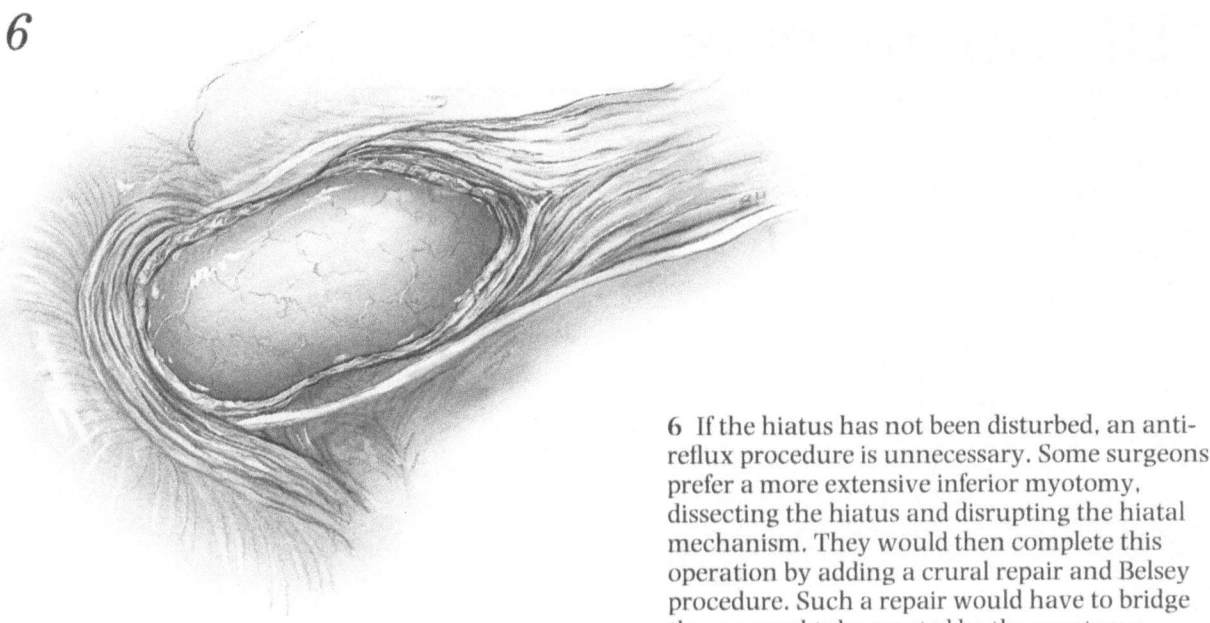

6 If the hiatus has not been disturbed, an anti-reflux procedure is unnecessary. Some surgeons prefer a more extensive inferior myotomy, dissecting the hiatus and disrupting the hiatal mechanism. They would then complete this operation by adding a crural repair and Belsey procedure. Such a repair would have to bridge the mucosal tube created by the myotomy.

Swallowing may commence with liquids on the first post-operative day, followed by soft diet and then normal food over the next 2–3 days.

18 Leiomyoma

These benign tumours occur within the muscular layers of the oesophagus. They may become large and lobulated or even cirsoid. The mucosa remains intact unless one ill-advisedly attempts endoscopic biopsy. Tumours within the lower oesophagus may be approached through a left thoracotomy, but those elsewhere within the thoracic oesophagus should be approached through a right thoracotomy at the level of the main tumour mass. A double-lumen tube will allow collapse of the ipsilateral lung, facilitating exposure.

The example illustrated below is of a leiomyoma arising at the level of the azygos vein. The surgical approach is by right thoracotomy through the bed of the fifth rib.

1

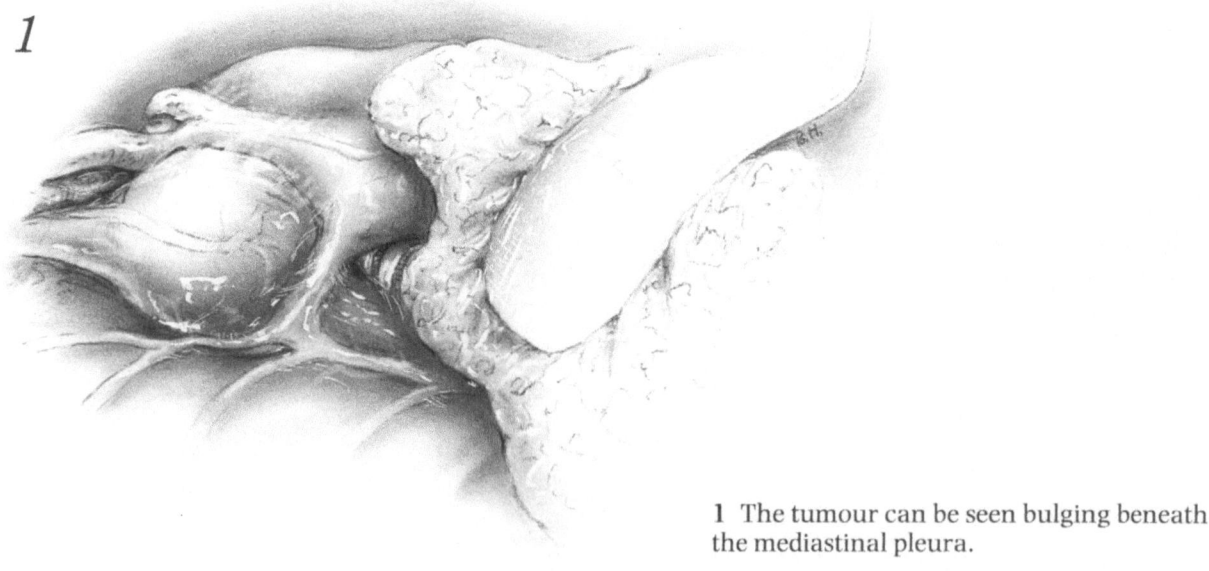

1 The tumour can be seen bulging beneath the mediastinal pleura.

2

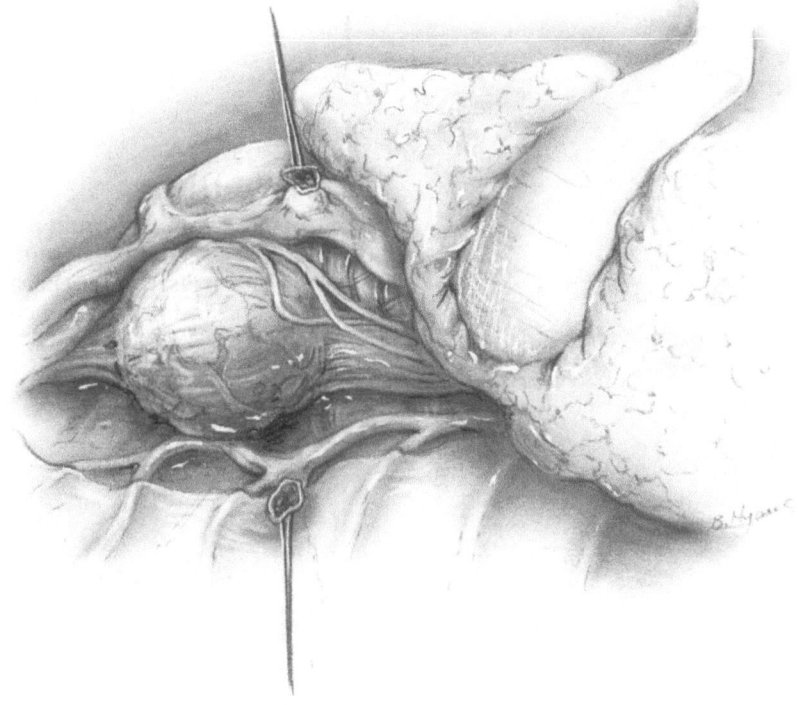

2 Division of the azygos vein allows exposure of the oesophagus from the diaphragmatic hiatus to the thoracic inlet. The branches of the vagus nerve can be seen passing over the surface of the tumour, which is still covered by thinned oesophageal muscle.

3

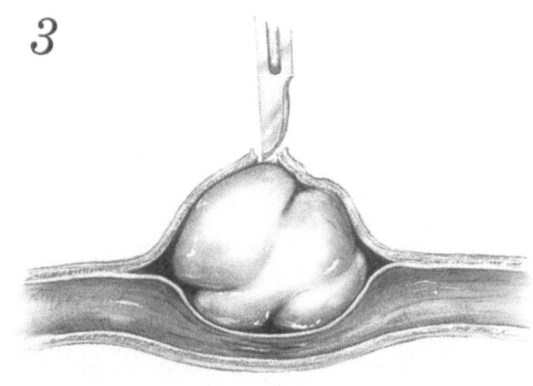

3 By rotation of the oesophagus one can usually discern on which side of the tumour lies the oesophageal lumen. This procedure may be helped by the passage of a nasogastric tube. A longitudinal myotomy is created over the tumour surface.

4

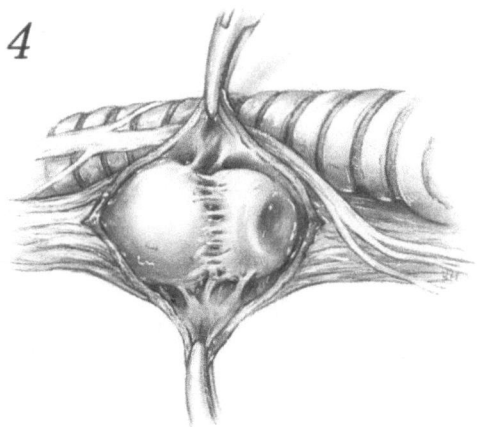

4 A plane of dissection readily develops between the normal oesophageal muscle and the underlying leiomyoma. The myotomy should be of sufficient length to permit ready delivery of these bulky tumours.

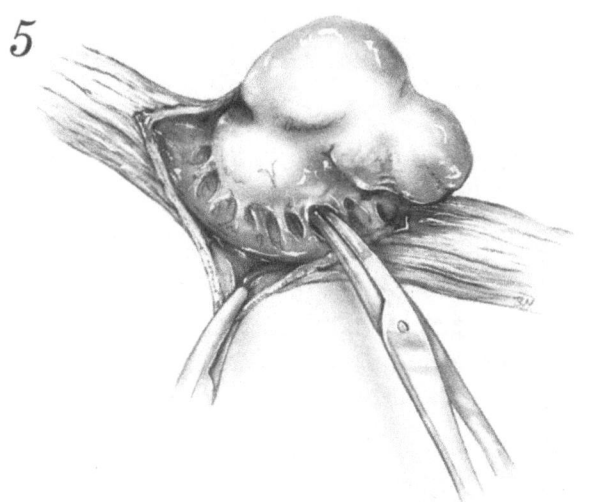

5 Blunt dissection continues over the surface of the tumour, which is lifted from the underlying mucosa. Sharp dissection separates it from the mucosal tube and perforation can usually be avoided.

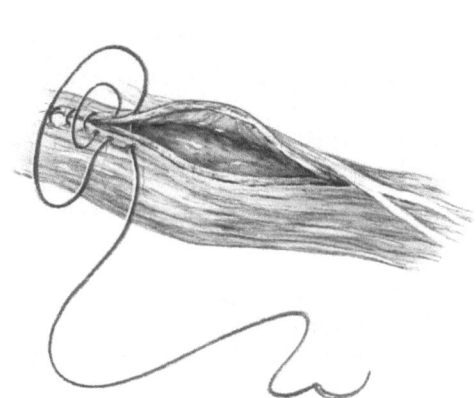

6 The muscle layer of the oesophagus is repaired with continuous monofilament non-absorbable suture.

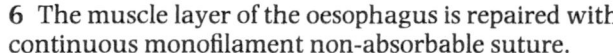

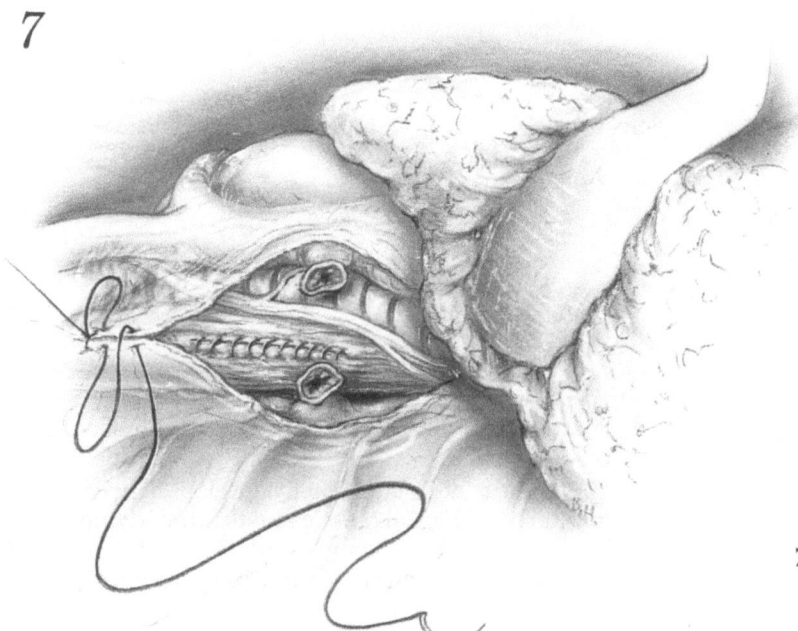

7 The mediastinal pleura is repaired.

The patient should commence fluid diet the following day. Early re-exploration is advised if there is any evidence to suggest an unsuspected perforation with oesophago-pleural fistula.

19 Carcinoma: Left-Sided Approach for Resection of the Lower Oesophagus and Gastro-oesophageal Junction (Logan Operation)

This extensive operation allows en bloc resection of the oesophagus and adjacent lymph nodes from the level of the carina, extending inferiorly to the coeliac axis. It is undertaken with curative intent and less ambitious resections should be used in patients clearly incurable. The proximal macroscopic extent of tumour as assessed endoscopically and on contrast X-rays must be beyond the lower margin of the aortic arch. At this level sufficient oesophagus can usually be devolved from beneath the aortic arch so as to permit an anastomosis below the aorta, but if additional length is required the oesophagus may be mobilised above the aorta and brought outwith the aortic arch.

Prophylactic antibiotics should be given for 24 hours to cover the aerobic and anaerobic organisms found in the obstructed oesophagus.

Intravenous crystalloids should be restricted during surgery, as any overload may add to postoperative respiratory difficulties.

An endobronchial tube passed by the anaesthetist will allow collapse of the left lung and facilitate dissection in the chest.

The left side of the neck should be left free of venous catheters in case the surgeon feels it desirable to take the anastomosis to the neck.

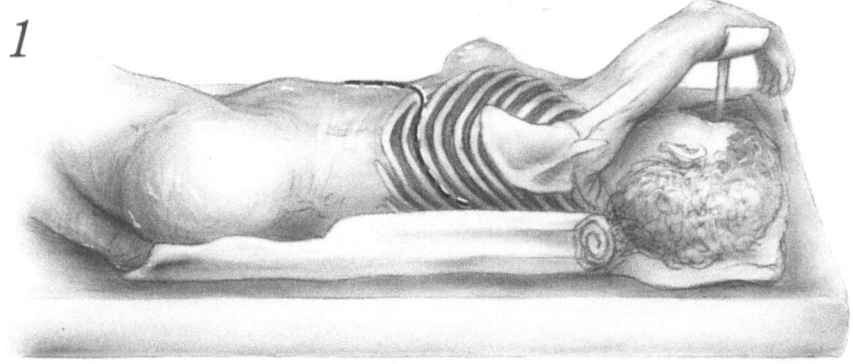

1 The patient is positioned in the left anterior oblique position with a support beneath the spine. The scapula is rotated from the operative field by supporting the arm on a rest above the head. A long oblique incision is made from the linea alba, midway between xiphoid and umbilicus, diagonally to the costal margin and along the line of the eighth rib beneath the tip of the scapula.

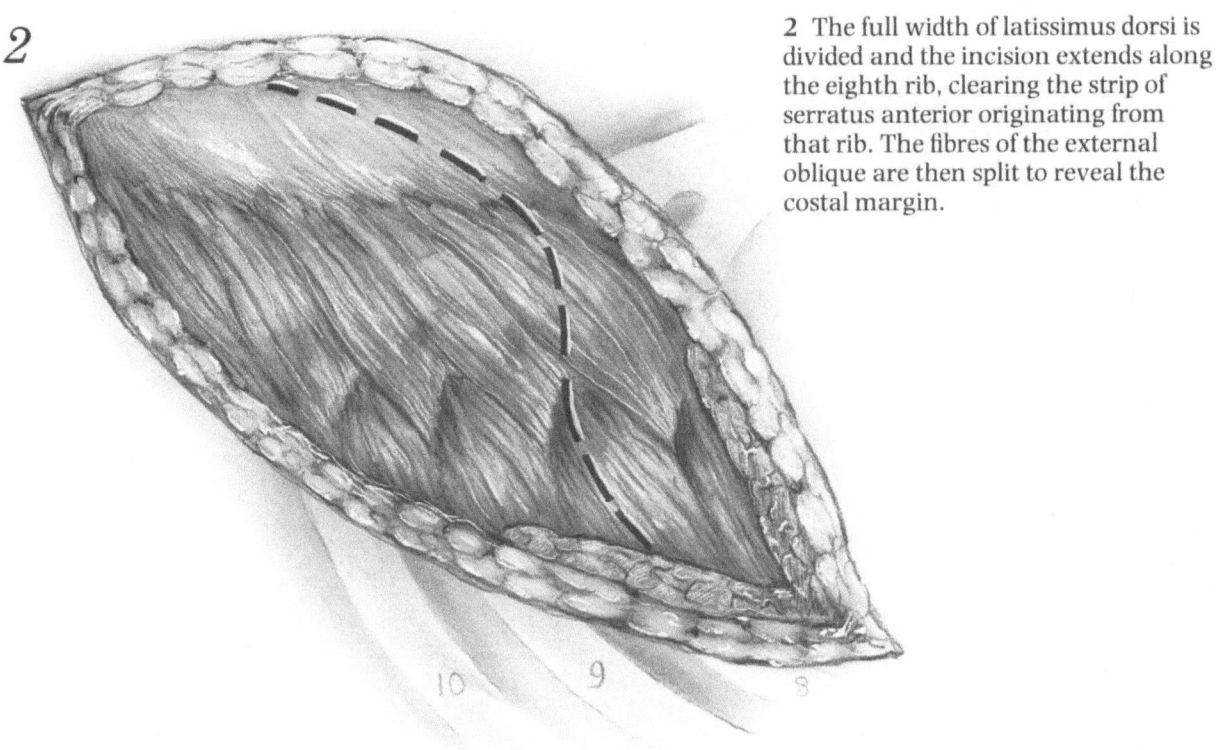

2 The full width of latissimus dorsi is divided and the incision extends along the eighth rib, clearing the strip of serratus anterior originating from that rib. The fibres of the external oblique are then split to reveal the costal margin.

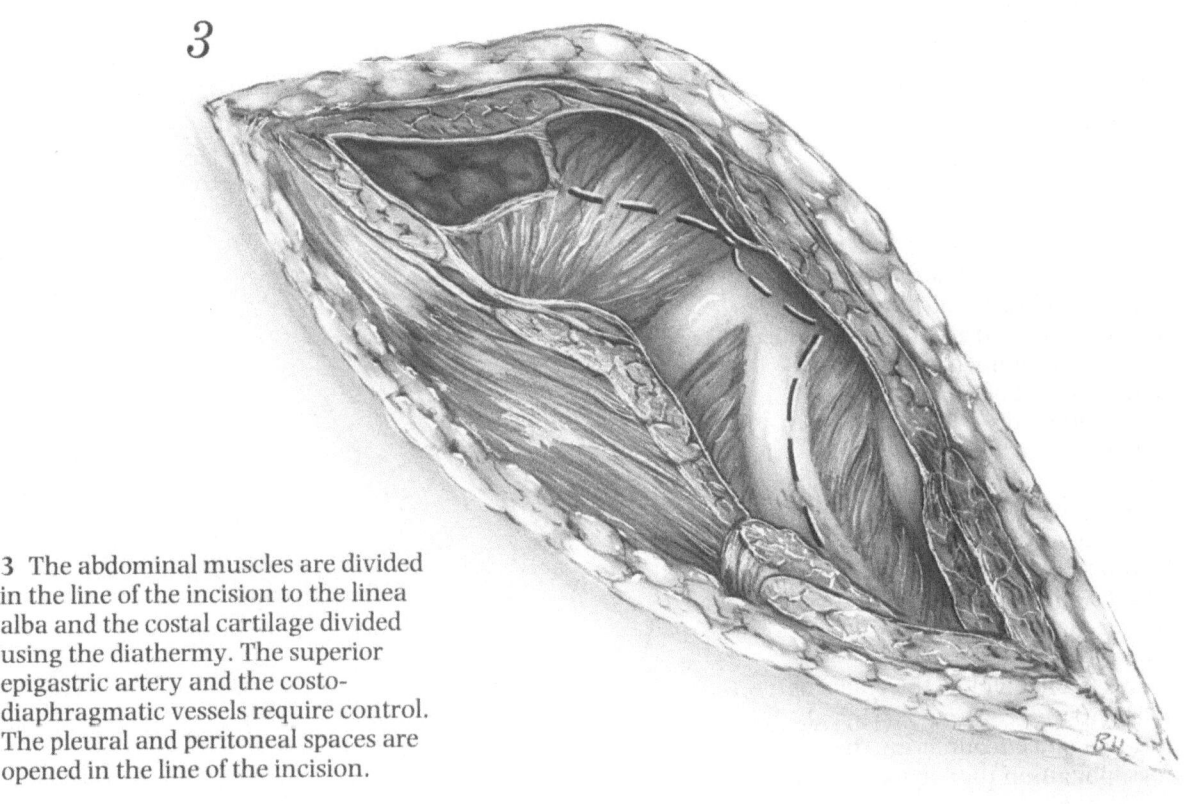

3 The abdominal muscles are divided in the line of the incision to the linea alba and the costal cartilage divided using the diathermy. The superior epigastric artery and the costo-diaphragmatic vessels require control. The pleural and peritoneal spaces are opened in the line of the incision.

4

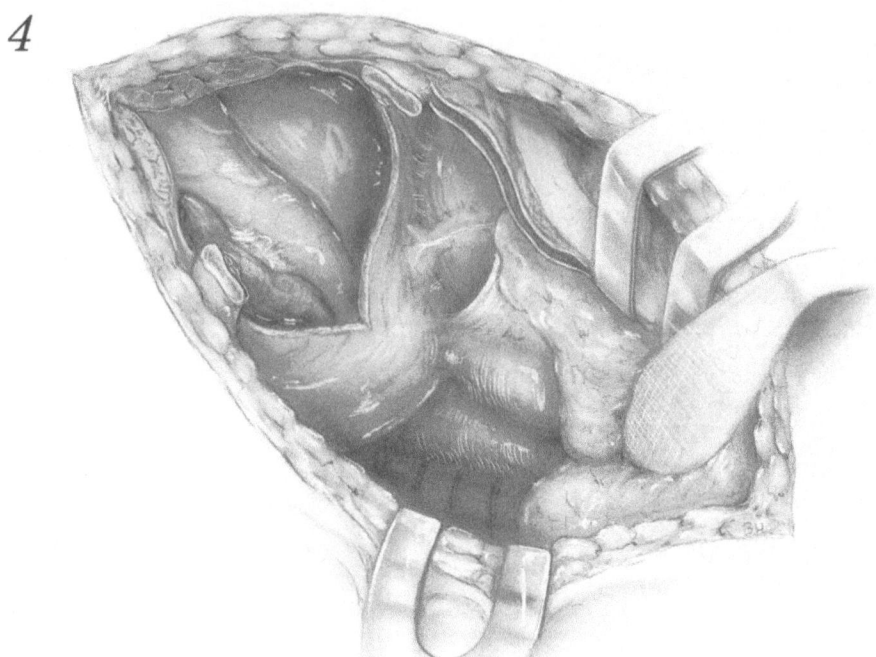

4 The diaphragm is divided beneath the costal margin, passing circumferentially to skirt the central tendon and then to spiral towards the oesophageal hiatus. In this way phrenic function is preserved to a large flap of the diaphragm whilst allowing the thoracic and abdominal dissections to be performed in continuity. A short length of the costal arch should be resected such that on closure the lower margin of the seventh rib abuts the upper margin of the eighth rib. Troublesome clicking of the costal arch may otherwise occur on movement.

5

5 The inferior pulmonary ligament is divided close to the lung surface and the lung retracted. Mediastinal dissection commences along the lateral aspect of the aorta. The adventitia is divided and reflected anteriorly to disclose the oesophageal branches of the aorta. These are divided between ligatures. Dissection proceeds inferiorly through the left crus of the diaphragm, allowing the hiatus to be reflected anteriorly. Dissection superiorly continues around the aortic arch, dividing the vagus nerve distal to the recurrent laryngeal branch and encountering the oesophagus in the subaortic fossa.

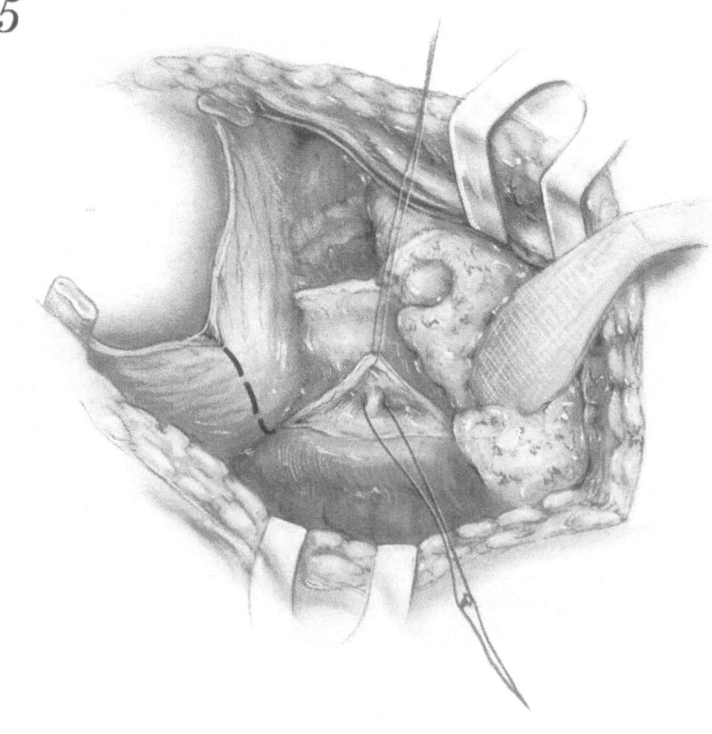

6

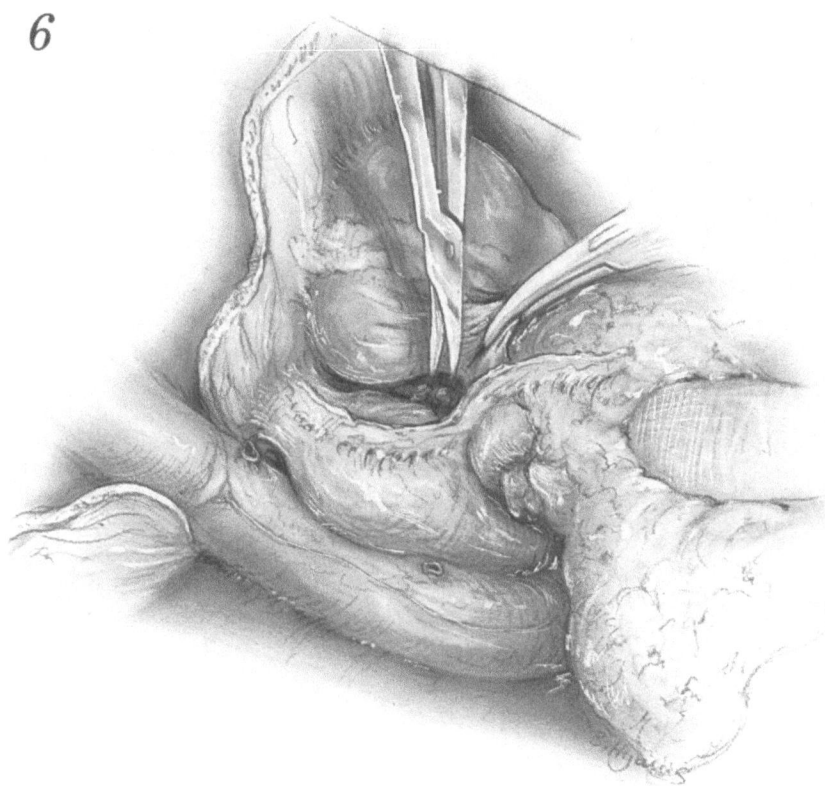

6 The anterior plane of mediastinal dissection is immediately posterior to the pericardium, reflecting mediastinal fat and the enclosed lymph nodes posteriorly onto the resection specimen. This dissection is carried superiorly, taking care in the region of the inferior pulmonary vein. The under-surface of the left main bronchus is identified and the main carinal lymph nodes are mobilised inferiorly onto the specimen. The anterior and posterior mediastinal dissection planes should then meet in the subaortic fossa.

7

7 The lieno-renal ligament is divided so that the spleen, the tail of the pancreas and the proximal stomach may be reflected to the right to reveal the left kidney, the adrenal and the lateral margin of the aorta.

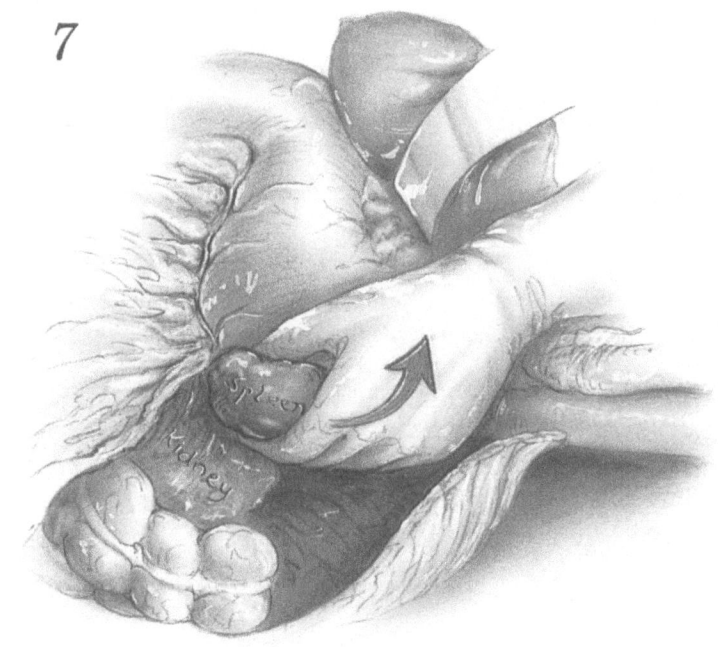

8

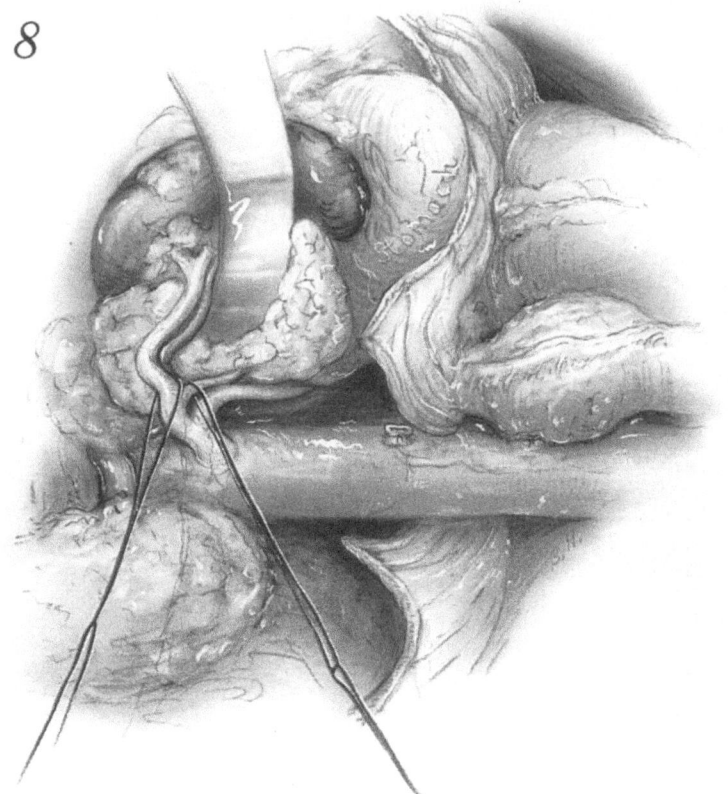

8 The mediastinal aortic dissection continues along the lateral surface of the abdominal aorta to the origin of the coeliac axis. The inferior phrenic vessels will be encountered and may be sacrificed. Many strands of nervous tissue within the coeliac plexus make this part of the dissection tedious and difficult. The root of the coeliac axis is identified and dissection continued along its branches until they can be clearly and unequivocally identified. Great care must be taken to preserve the hepatic artery which provides the blood supply to the gastric pedicle. The splenic artery and left gastric artery are doubly ligated at their origin and divided.

9

9 The body of the pancreas can then be reflected medially. The junction of the splenic and superior mesenteric veins is identified and the splenic vein divided. The pancreas is transected at this point. The pancreatic duct, if identified, should be transfixed and the pancreatic stump oversewn with a continuous soluble suture.

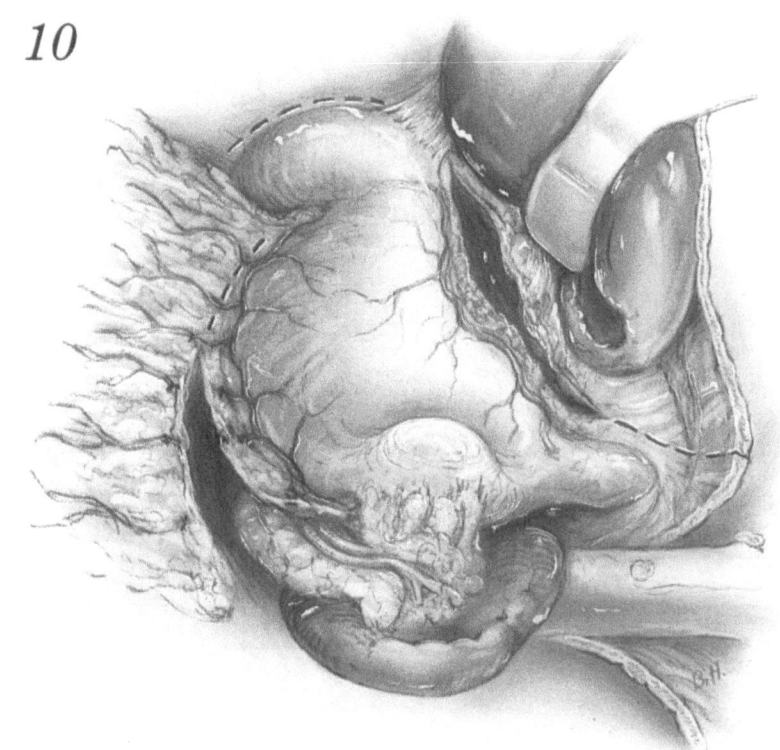

10 Mobilisation of the stomach proceeds along the greater omentum outwith the gastro-epiploeic vascular arcade. In ligating the epiploeic branches of this arcade, care must be taken to avoid the parent vessels, on which the viability of the stomach pedicle depends. Dissection along the greater curve proceeds to the entry of the right gastro-epiploeic artery, which is preserved. Dissection along the lesser curve is performed by dividing the lesser omentum. A Kocher manoeuvre is performed.

Mobilisation of the stomach and oesophagus is completed by dividing the right crus of the diaphragm. Dissection in this plane is carried superiorly, entering the right pleura. Care should be taken in identifying the azygos vein. The resection specimen is dissected from the right inferior pulmonary ligament. A pyloroplasty or pyloromyotomy is necessary only if the pylorus is scarred by coincident ulceration.

11

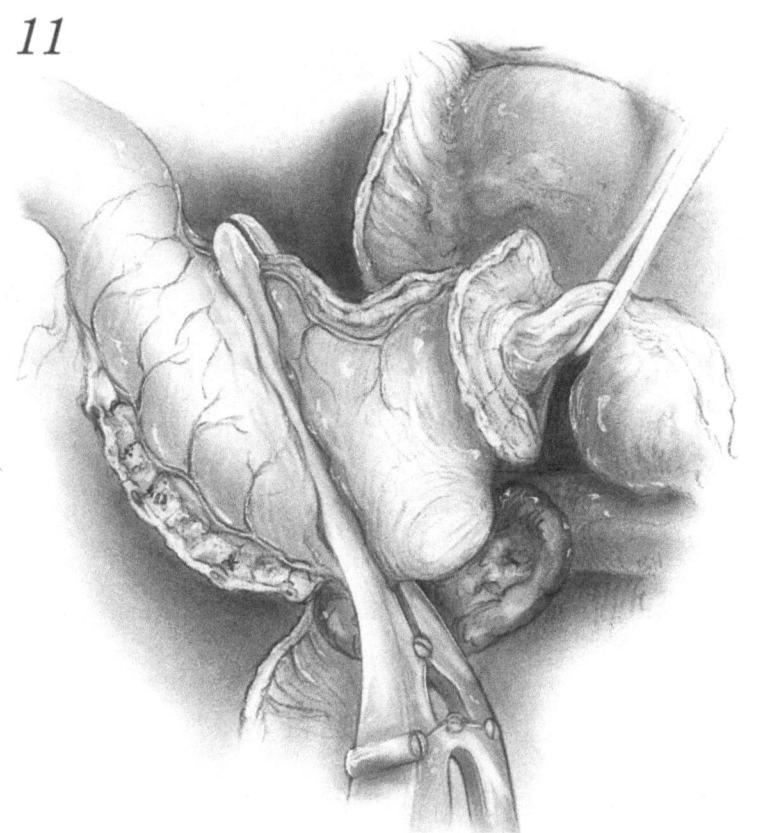

11 The gastric tube is fashioned, dividing the stomach obliquely with a Peyr's clamp. As much of the greater curve as possible should be preserved to provide length for the gastric tube. The transection of the lesser curve should pass distal to the insertion of the left gastric artery, leaving all glands on the resection specimen.

12

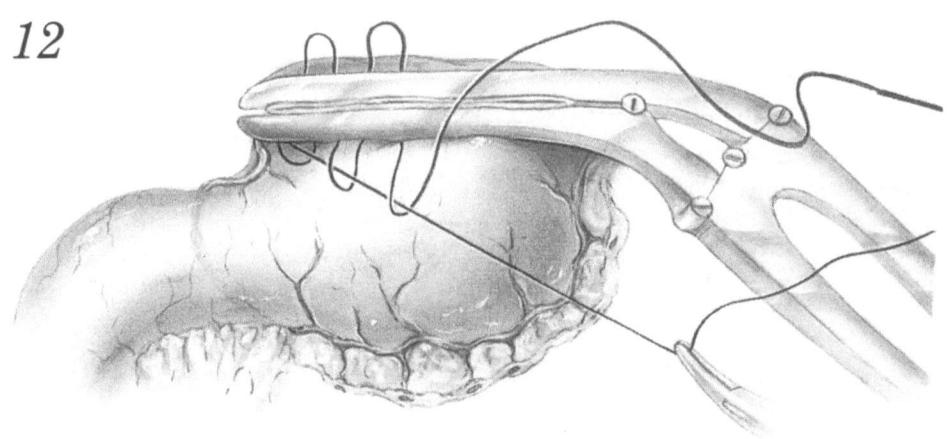

12 The stomach is closed with a sewing machine suture of absorbable material. The illustration shows this suture in an exploded form—in reality it is necessary to maintain tension on the running suture.

13

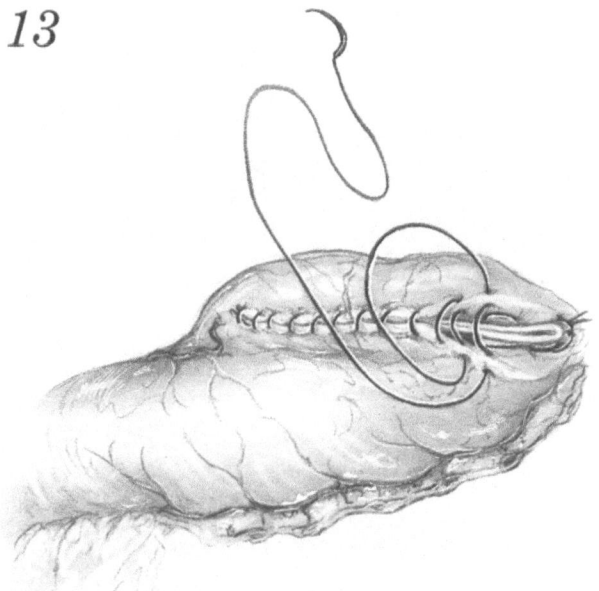

13 The crushed flange is inverted with a continuous non-absorbable suture.

14

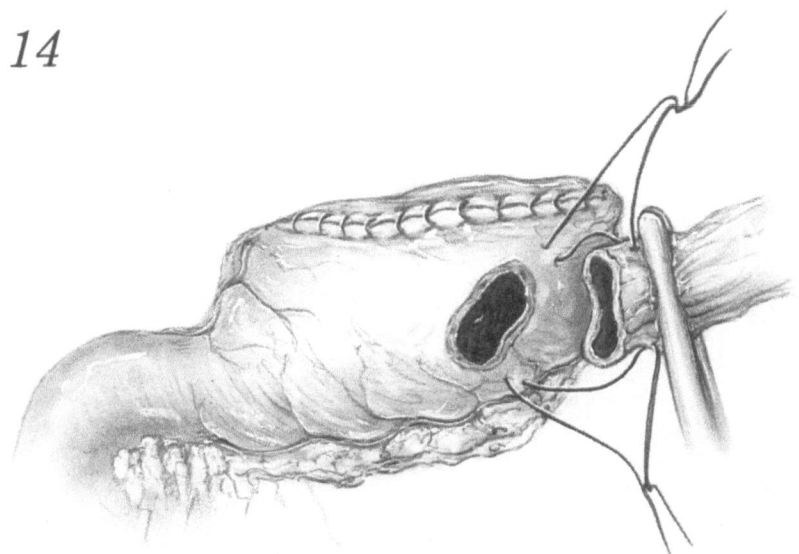

14 The oesophagus is divided at least 5 cm above the macroscopic limit of the tumour. A light occlusion clamp across the proximal oesophagus prevents spill of stagnant oesophageal contents and allows gentle traction during the anastomosis. The gastric tube is laid into the mediastinal bed and a suitable site is selected on the anterior wall of the stomach, well away from the gastro-epiploeic arcade and the stomach closure. A full thickness disc of the stomach is excised. Careful haemostasis may be necessary if profuse bleeding is encountered from the submucosal vessels. The stomach is brought to the oesophagus with stay sutures.

15

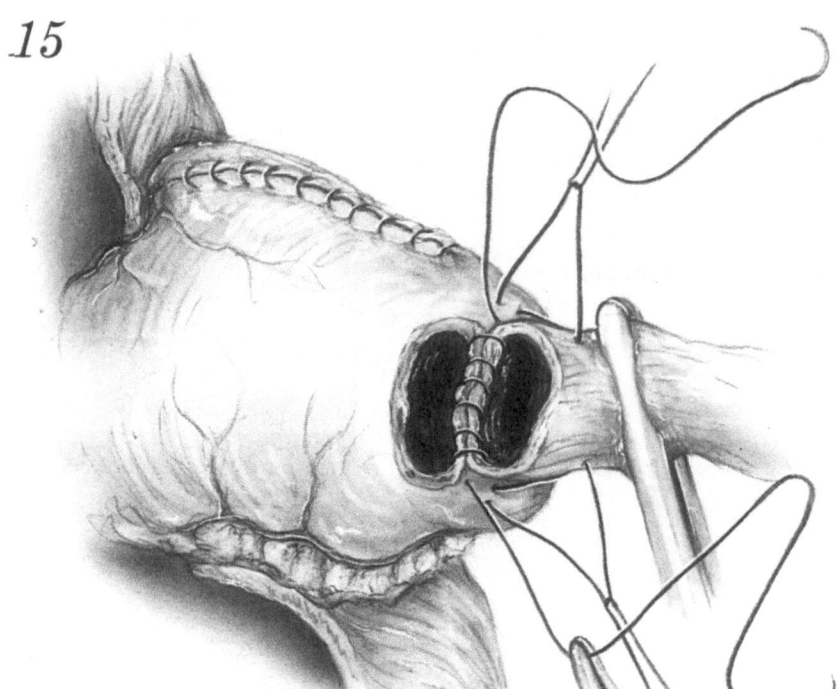

15 An end to side oesophago-gastric anastomosis is then performed using a continuous suture of 3.0 monofilament non-absorbable suture. If a nasogastric tube is required post-operatively it may be passed across the anastomosis at this stage, before completion.

16

16 The anastomosis is invaginated into the gastric tube using interrupted non-absorbable sutures.

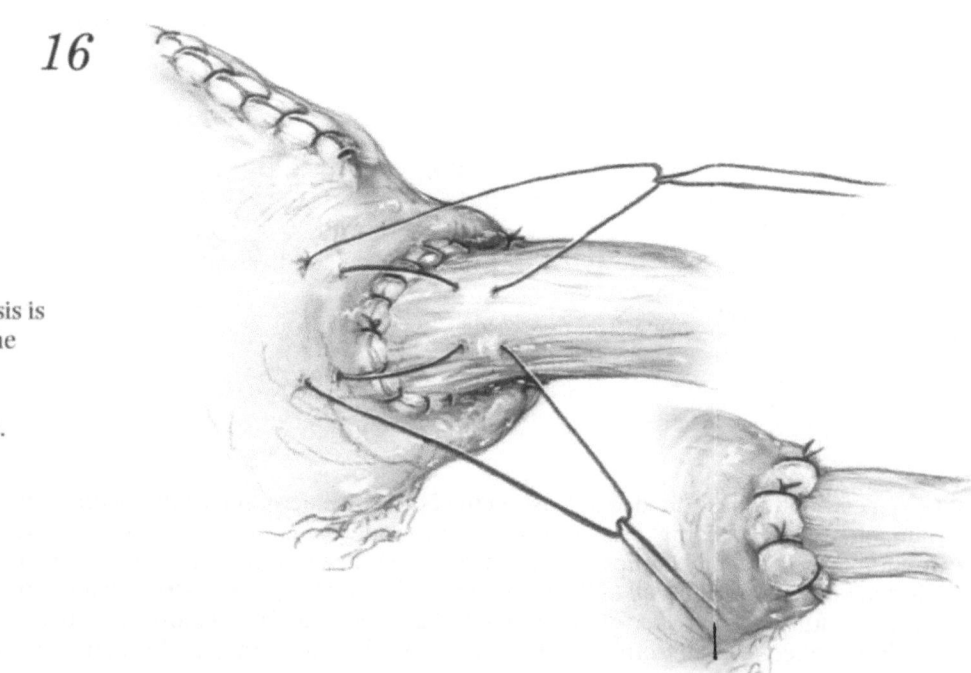

17

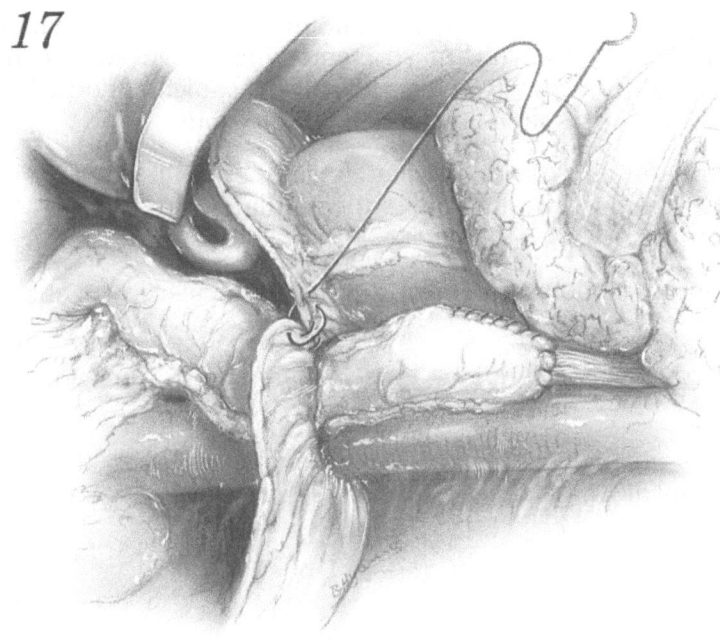

17 The anastomosis should lie within the mediastinum without tension. The diaphragm is repaired with a continuous suture of soluble material. The margins of the gastric tube are sutured to the new hiatus with interrupted sutures.

18

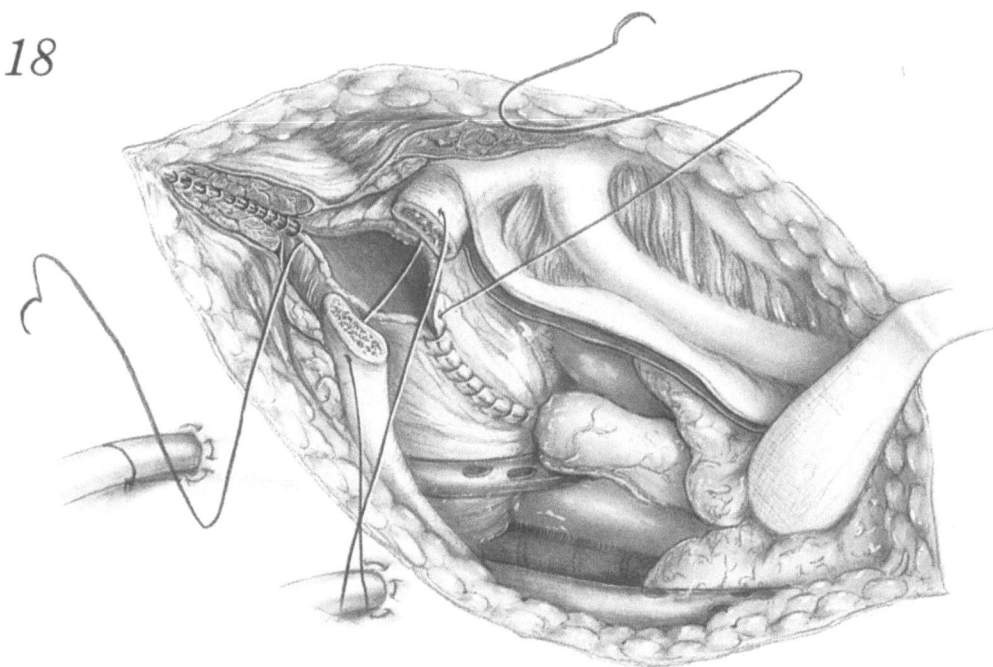

18 Closure of the diaphragm continues on to the posterior oblique muscles. Two chest drains are required, one of which passes across the mediastinum to drain the right pleural space. The ribs and costal margin are approximated using interrupted sutures. The muscles of the chest and abdominal walls are then closed in layers.

Free reflux will occur after this operation and fatal aspiration pneumonia may result. The patient should remain 30° head up at all times, especially whilst gastric emptying is delayed. It is my practice to return the patient to the ward from theatre with the inflated cuffed endotracheal tube in place. It is only removed once the patient is semi-erect and fully conscious.

This operation may take several hours and as a result the patient may be cold and acidotic. It is often preferable to undertake a few hours of positive pressure ventilation to allow cardio-vascular and biochemical homeostasis.

Intravenous fluid restriction should continue following surgery and volume replacement should be undertaken with colloid and blood.

Respiratory difficulties are common after this operation, especially amongst smokers, and vigorous physiotherapy is essential.

Ileus is uncommon, and gastric emptying usually resumes 2–3 days after surgery. At this time oral fluids may be commenced and normal diet introduced over successive days.

20 Carcinoma: Oesophageal Resection from the Right (McKeown Operation)

This is the preferred approach for tumours of the oesophagus at or above the aortic arch. It is a three-stage operation: (a) midline laparotomy to mobilise the stomach and hiatus, allowing assessment of intra-abdominal metastases; (b) right thoracotomy to mobilise the oesophagus and tumour; and (c) a cervical incision to perform the anastomosis. The third step may be omitted and an intra-thoracic anastomosis undertaken (Ivor Lewis operation). However, if the anastomosis is within the chest the consequences of anastomotic leak are disastrous and there is some evidence to suggest that such anastomoses are associated with more troublesome reflux problems.

Prophylactic antibiotics should be given for 24 hours to cover the aerobic and anaerobic organisms found in the obstructed oesophagus.

Intravenous crystalloids should be restricted during surgery, as any overload may add to post-operative respiratory difficulties.

An endobronchial tube passed by the anaesthetist will allow the collapse of the right lung and facilitate dissection in the chest.

The operative side of the neck should be left free of venous catheters.

1

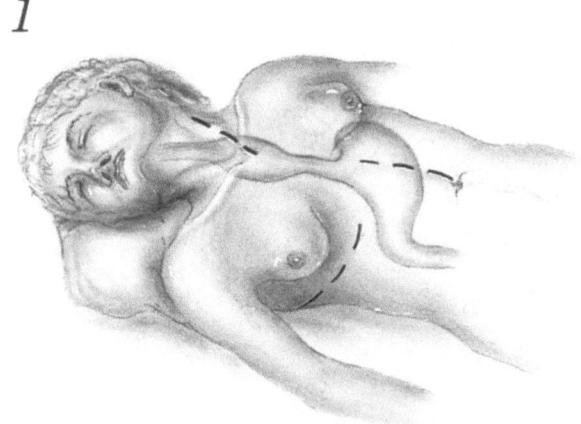

1 It is possible to position the patient so that all three incisions may be performed without re-draping. This is not the author's practice and it is not recommended for those unfamiliar with the operation. The patient is positioned supine for the abdominal incision. Once this stage is completed the patient is turned into the lateral position, re-draped and the thoracotomy stage undertaken. At the end of the second stage the patient is placed supine with the neck slightly flexed and rotated to the dominant side, and the third stage performed through a cervical incision on the non-dominant side.

2 A midline epigastric incision is performed from the xiphoid process, stopping short of the umbilicus. The incision is deepened through the linea alba and the peritoneum is opened. The liver may be palpated for metastases and this may be facilitated by division of the falciform ligament. The left lobe of the liver is mobilised by division of the triangular ligament and the coeliac axis may then be examined for the presence of fixed lymph nodes which may hamper dissection. The pylorus should be inspected for coincident ulceration or scarring.

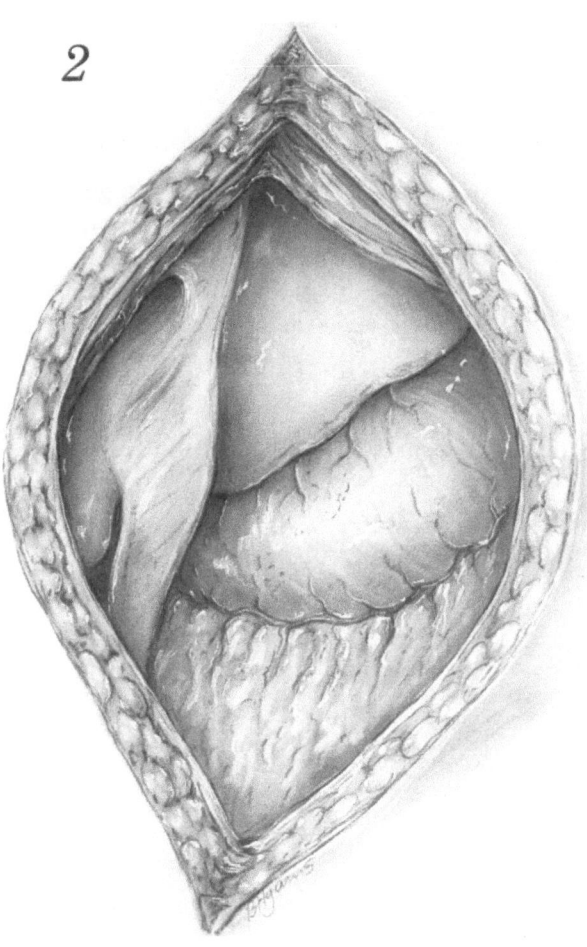

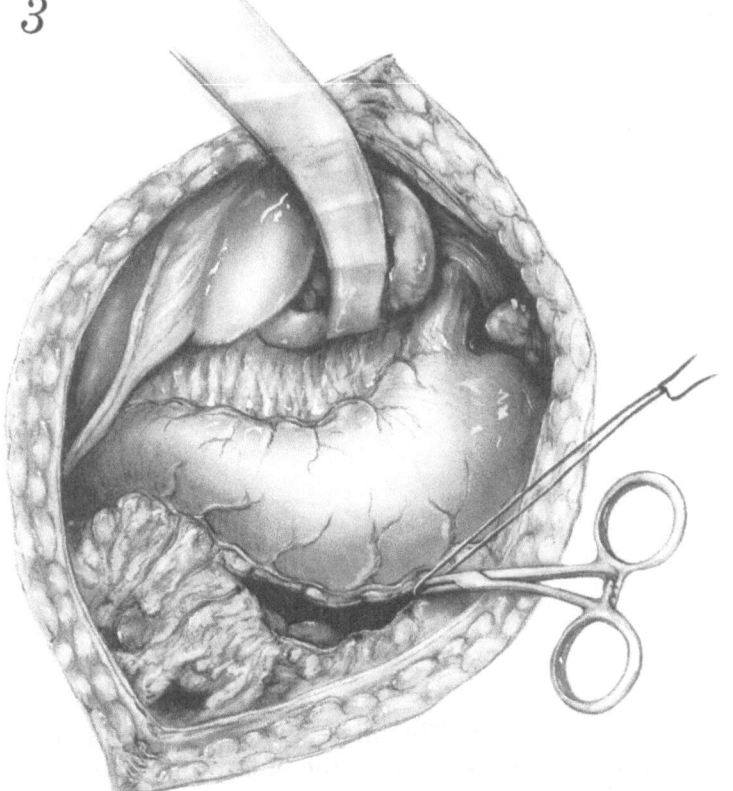

3 Mobilisation is commenced at the midpoint of the greater curve by dividing the greater omentum outwith the gastro-epiploeic arcades. In tying the epiploeic branches of this arcade, care must be taken not to injure the gastro-epiploeic arterial arcade on which the vascularity of the stomach and anastomosis depends. Mobilisation should continue distally along the gastro-epiploeic arcade to the entry of the right gastro-epiploeic artery, which must be preserved. Mobilisation continues proximally along the greater curve, dividing the left gastro-epiploeic artery.

4

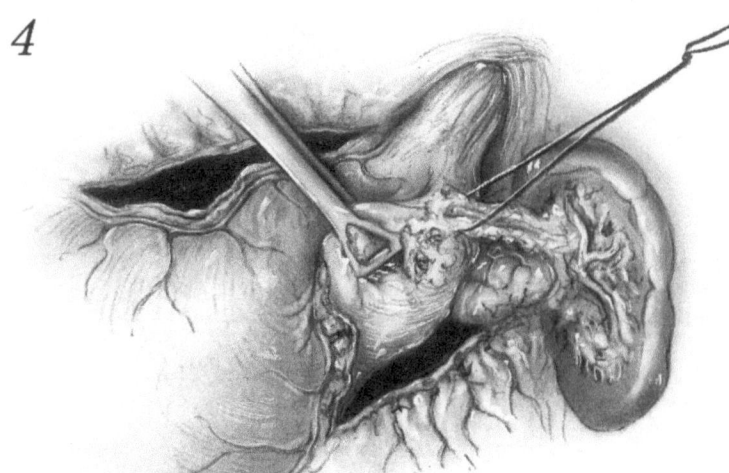

4 The short gastric arteries are identified and divided, taking care not to include the stomach wall. This mobilisation may be facilitated by rotating the operating table towards the patient's right and by drawing the fundus of the stomach inferiorly with a tissue forcep. Mobilisation should now be complete to the oesophageal hiatus. Mobilisation along the lesser curve divides the lesser omentum, taking care to identify any aberrant hepatic branches of the left gastric artery.

5

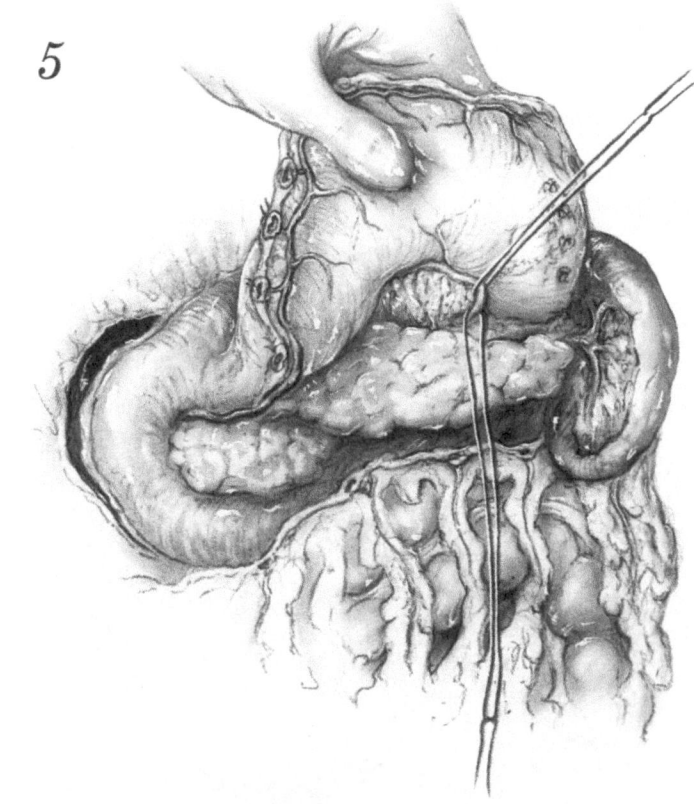

5 The mobilised stomach may now be lifted upwards, to identify the left gastric artery as it emerges from the upper border of the pancreas. It should be divided as close to the retroperitoneal wall as possible and double ligatures are recommended on this large, often atheromatous vessel. If the pylorus is normal there is no need for a pyloroplasty or pyloromyotomy.

The abdominal closure commences with the peritoneum. The linea alba is closed using a continuous monofilament non-absorbable suture, taking care to bury the bulky knots. The closure is then completed by subcutaneous and skin closure.

6

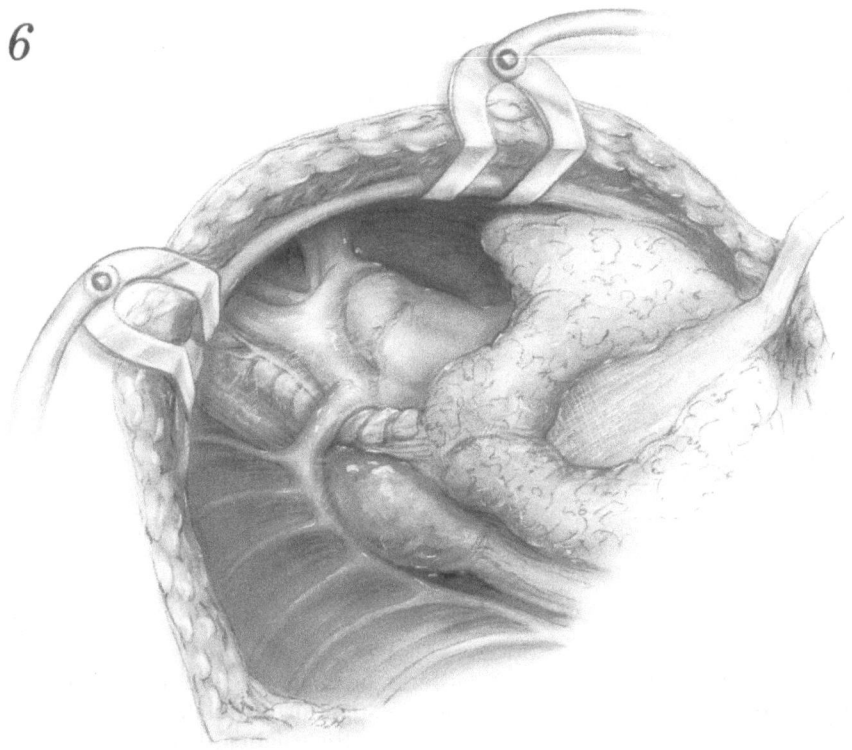

6 A right lateral thoracotomy is undertaken through the bed of the sixth rib. The lung is retracted anteriorly and this may be facilitated by a double-lumen endobronchial tube which allows collapse of the right lung. The inferior pulmonary ligament is mobilised close to the lung surface.

7

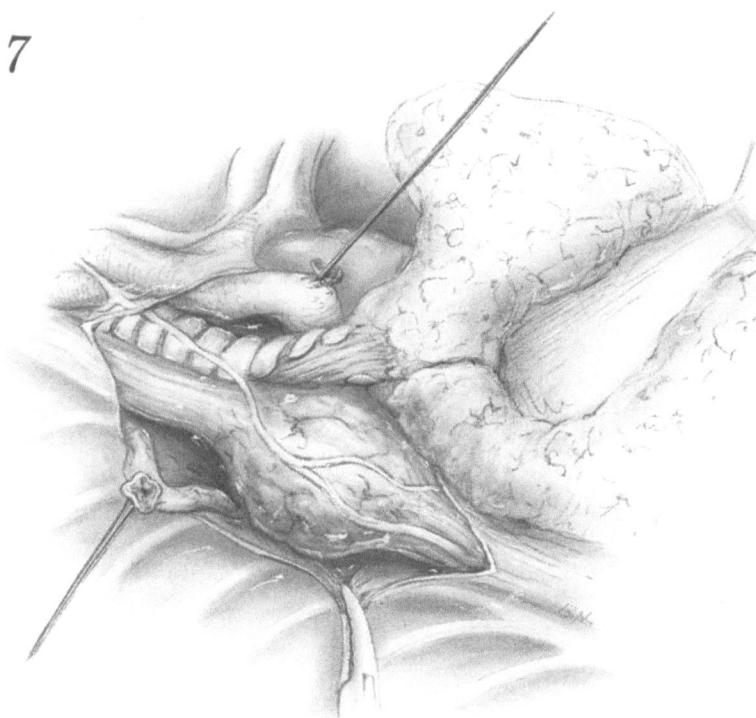

7 The mediastinal pleura is opened along the lateral aspect of the oesophagus. Division of the azygos arch then allows access to the whole length of the intra-thoracic oesophagus. If the tumour is adherent a segment of the vein may be left attached.

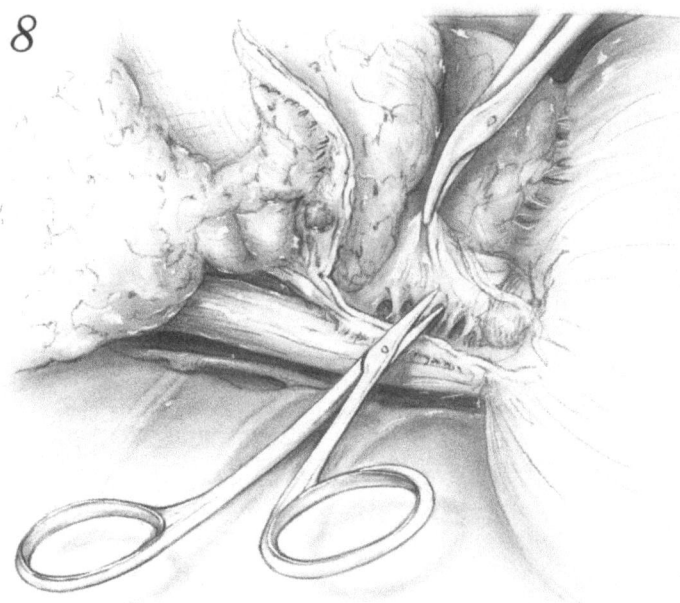

8 The anterior dissection plane is commenced behind the pericardium. It progresses inferiorly to link with the hiatal dissection from the laparotomy incision. Dissection is carried superiorly, mobilising the oesophagus and tumour from the back of the right pulmonary hilum and the trachea. The main carinal lymph nodes should be dissected onto the resection specimen. The posterior resection plane is immediately anterior to the azygos vein; it continues cephalad along the vein and above the azygos arch to the thoracic inlet. The thoracic duct may be identified anywhere along its intra-thoracic course. It is most at risk low in the chest lying between the azygos vein and aorta or at mid-thoracic level, where it crosses behind the oesophagus to the left.

9

9 With traction on the upper thoracic oesophagus blunt dissection can be continued along the oesophagus into the root of the neck. The right recurrent laryngeal nerve is frequently seen looping beneath the subclavian artery.

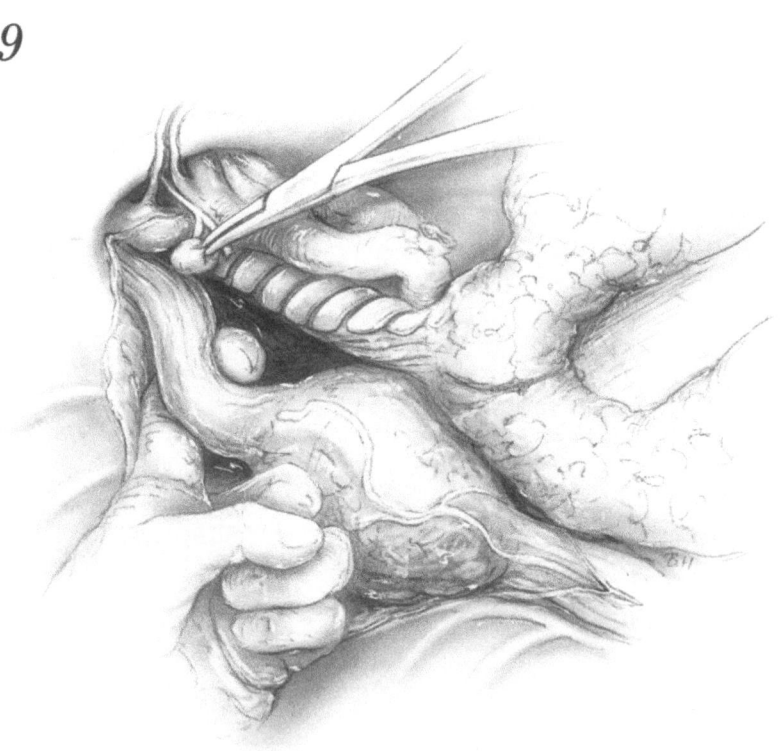

10

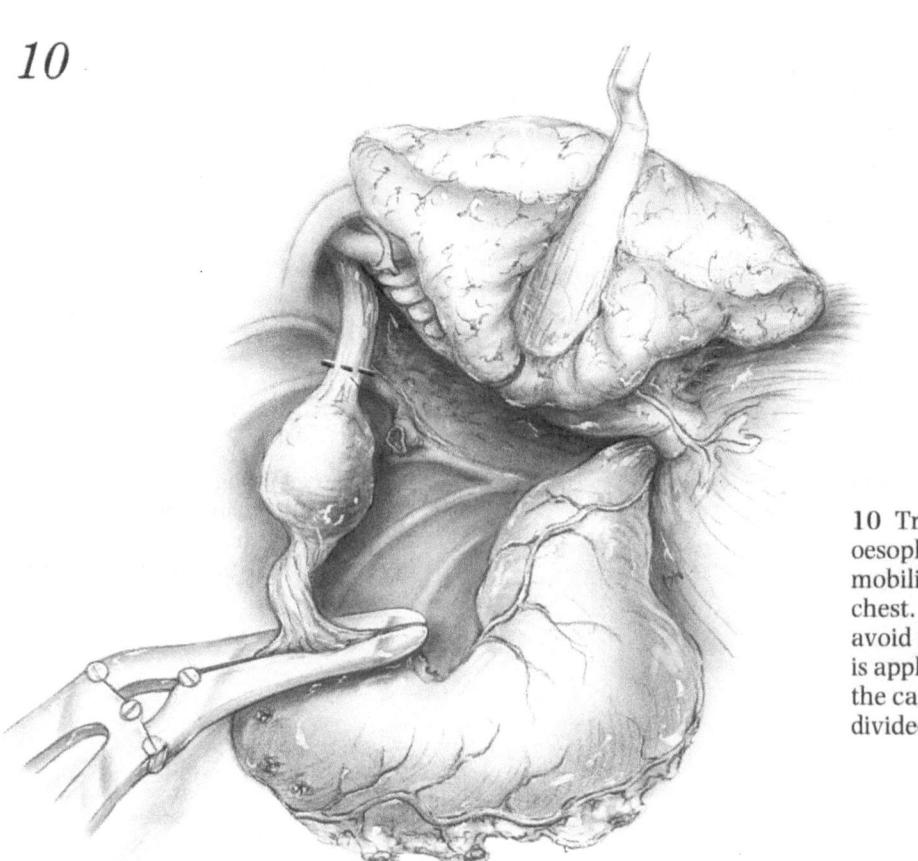

10 Traction on the lower oesophagus delivers the mobilised stomach into the chest. Care should be taken to avoid rotation. A Peyr's clamps is applied on the gastric side of the cardia, and the stomach divided.

11

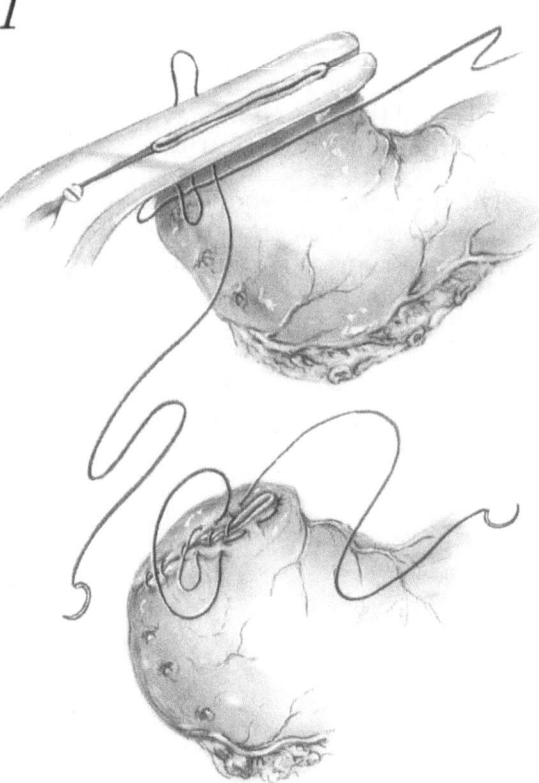

11 The stomach is closed with a continuous sewing machine suture of absorbable material and the crush flange is inverted with an over and over suture of non-absorbable material. The redundant oesophagus containing the tumour is excised.

12

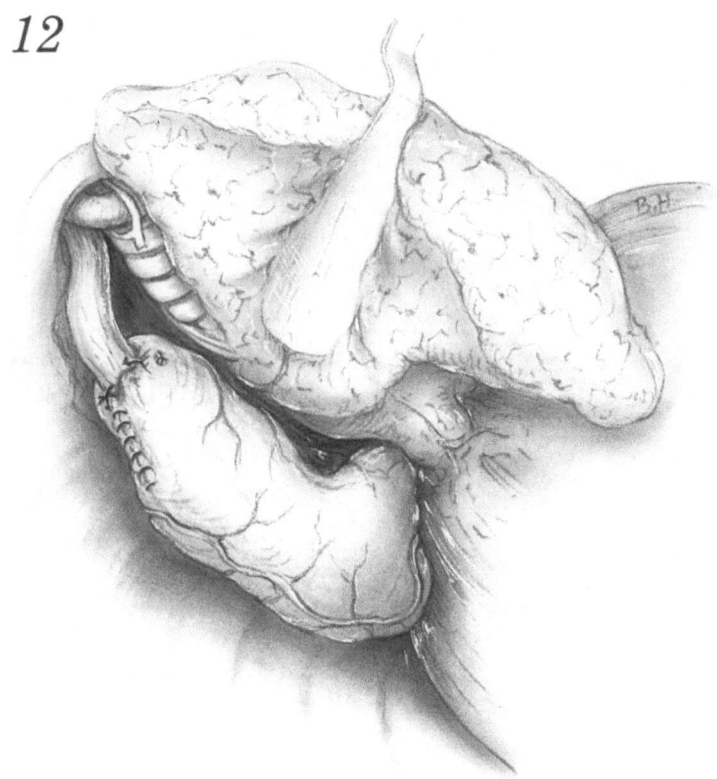

12 The oesophageal stump is loosely tacked to the gastric tube at the site of the proposed anastomosis. This should be well away from the gastric closure.

If desired the operation may end at this point by performing an intra-thoracic oesophago-gastric anastomosis (see Chap. 19).

The thoracotomy wound is closed after inserting a chest drain. The ribs are approximated using interrupted strong non-absorbable sutures and the rest of the wound closed in layers using continuous sutures of absorbable material.

13 The neck incision is then performed on the left, passing along the anterior border of the sternomastoid muscle. The dissection proceeds medial to the carotid sheath, dividing the middle thyroid vein and omohyoid muscle.

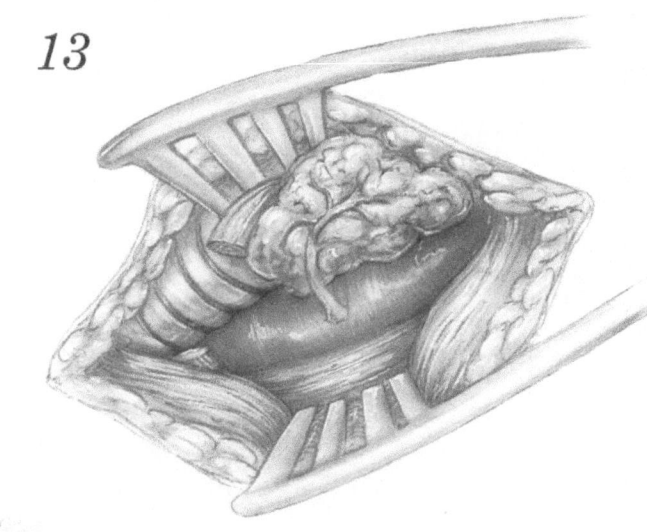

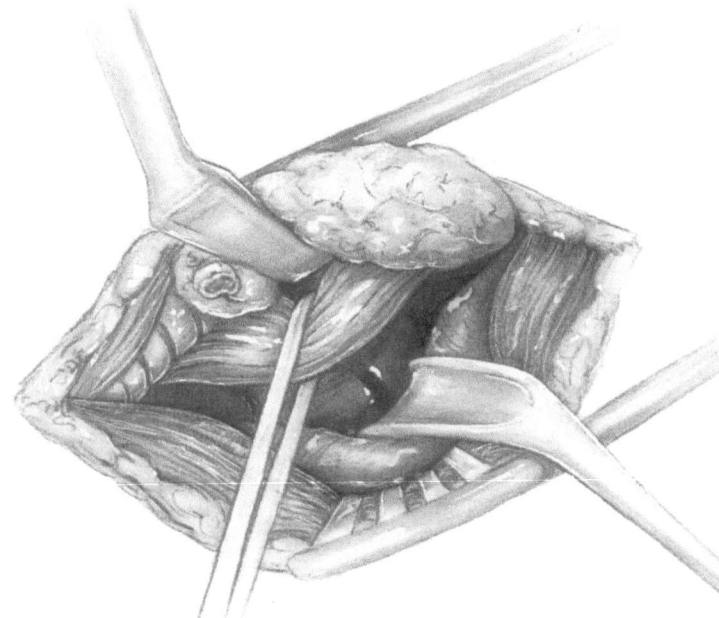

14 The oesophagus is identified, lying between the trachea and the prevertebral fascia. This dissection is facilitated by the mobilisation begun within the chest. The ipsilateral recurrent laryngeal nerve should be identified and a sling passed around the oesophagus, keeping close to its wall in an effort to avoid the contralateral recurrent laryngeal nerve.

15 Traction on the cervical oesophagus will then deliver the gastric tube into the neck. The oesophageal remnant is then detached from the stomach and the definitive site of oesophageal transection is selected. Oblique division of the oesophagus permits a wider stoma and allows the anastomosis to sit comfortably on the anterior surface of the gastric tube.

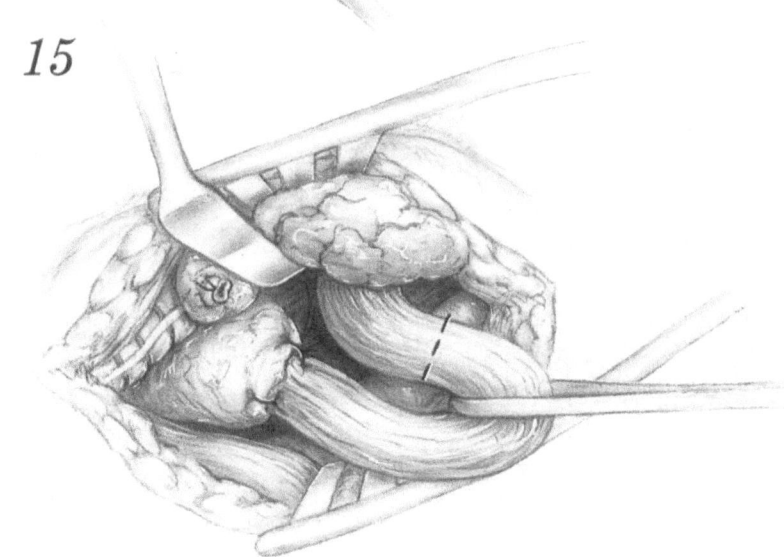

16

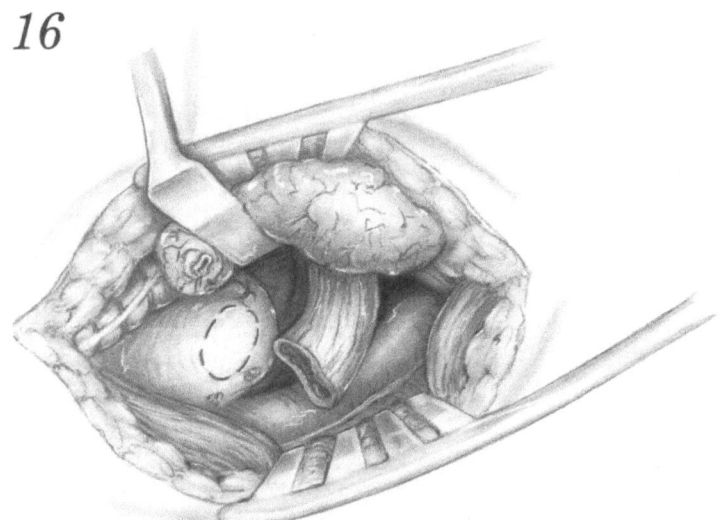

16 A suitable site for the anastomosis is identified on the fundus of stomach. A circular full thickness defect is created in the stomach, keeping away from the gastric closure. The submucosal plexus should bleed profusely and pinpoint haemostasis may be desirable. It is best not to attempt complete haemostasis and the anastomosis may be performed with some continued bleeding.

17

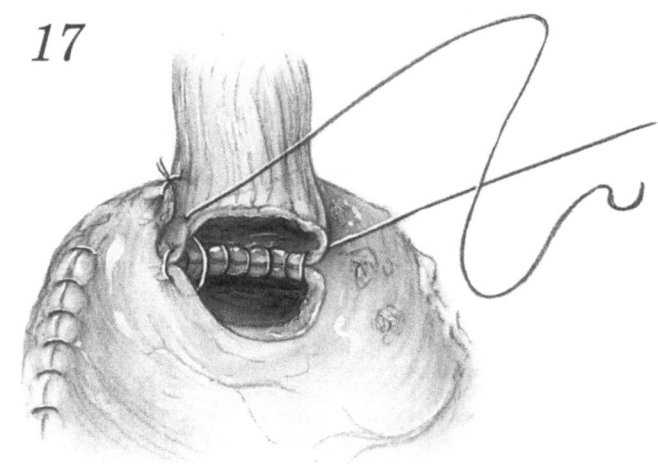

17 An end to side oesophago-gastric anastomosis is undertaken, using a single layer of continuous 3·0 monofilament non-absorbable suture, taking generous full thickness bites of oesophagus and stomach. If a nasogastric tube is required, it may be passed at this stage and negotiated into the stomach before the anastomosis is completed. The anastomosis may be facilitated by flexing the neck.

18

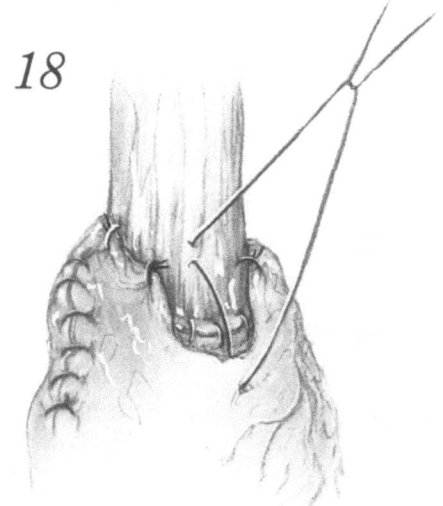

18 The anastomosis may be inverted into the gastric tube with interrupted non-absorbable sutures.

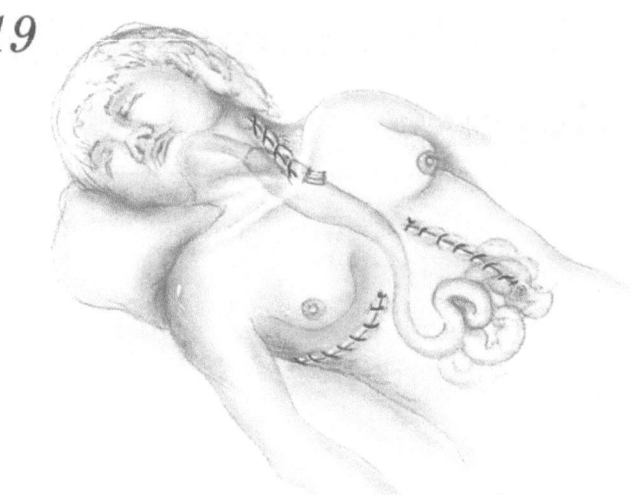

19 Before closing the cervical incision a corrugated drain is led from the region of the anastomosis through a separate stab incision. The wound is then closed in layers using continuous sutures of absorbable material.

Free reflux will occur after this operation and fatal aspiration pneumonia may result. The patient should remain 30° head up at all times, especially whilst gastric emptying is delayed. It is my practice to return the patient to the ward from theatre with the inflated cuffed endotracheal tube in place. It is only removed once the patient is semi-erect and fully conscious.

This operation may take several hours, and as a result the patient may be cold and acidotic. It is often preferable to undertake a few hours of positive pressure ventilation to allow cardio-vascular and biochemical haemostasis.

Intravenous fluid restriction should continue following surgery and volume replacement should be undertaken with colloid and blood.

Respiratory difficulties are common after this operation, especially amongst smokers, and vigorous physiotherapy is essential.

Ileus is uncommon, and gastric emptying usually resumes 2–3 days after surgery. At this time oral fluids may be commenced and normal diet introduced over successive days.

21 Carcinoma: Substernal Gastric Bypass

This operation is gaining increasing popularity to restore normal swallowing in patients with irresectable tumours of the thoracic portion of the oesophagus or in those not sufficiently fit to permit the extensive resection. It is particularly useful where tumours of the intra-thoracic oesophagus have eroded into adjacent organs such as lung, pleura or the tracheo-bronchial tree. Patients are not suitable if tumour or involved lymph nodes involve the cervical oesophagus or if there is involvement of the proximal stomach.

The approach is in many ways similar to trans-hiatal blunt oesophagectomy and the surgeon may approach the operation with this in mind, settling for a bypass should the tumour not prove readily resectable by blunt trans-hiatal dissection.

Prophylactic antibiotics are commenced with the premedication and given intravenously for 24 hours. The agents chosen should be effective against aerobic and anaerobic organisms usually encountered in the obstructed oesophagus.

1

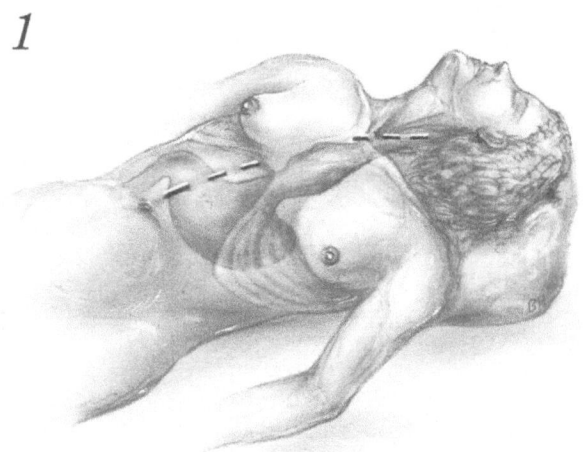

1 The patient is positioned supine, with the shoulders supported so that the neck may be extended. At a later stage it may be necessary to flex the neck to facilitate the anastomosis. The neck incision is performed on the side of the non-dominant arm and the head is rotated slightly away from the operative side. Any neck lines required for fluid or monitoring should be inserted in the contralateral subclavian or jugular veins.

2 A midline epigastric incision is performed from the xiphoid process, stopping short of the umbilicus. The incision is deepened through the linea alba and the peritoneum is opened. The liver may be palpated for metastases and this may be facilitated by division of the falciform ligament. The left lobe of the liver is mobilised by division of the triangular ligament and the coeliac axis may then be examined for the presence of fixed lymph nodes which may hamper dissection. The pylorus should be inspected for coincident ulceration or scarring.

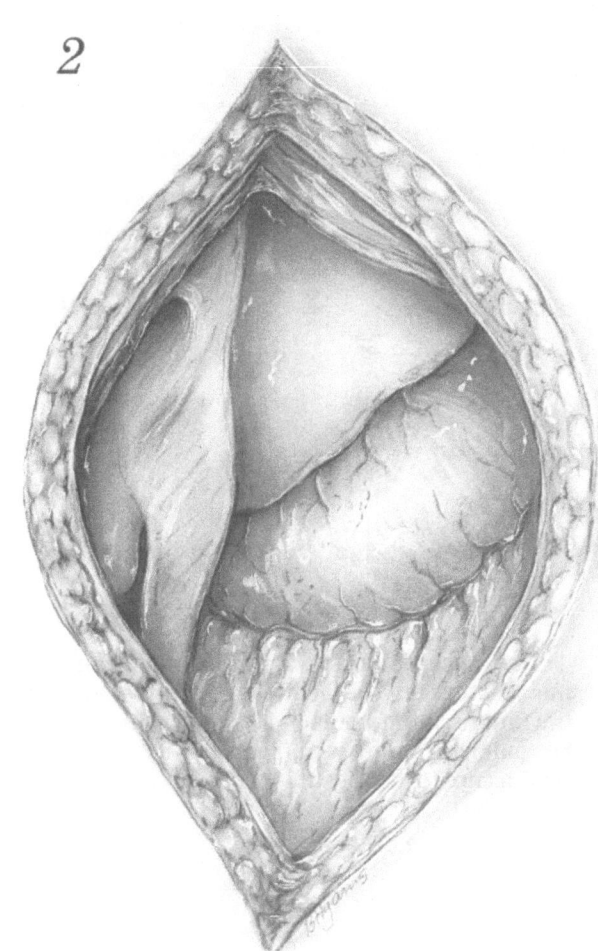

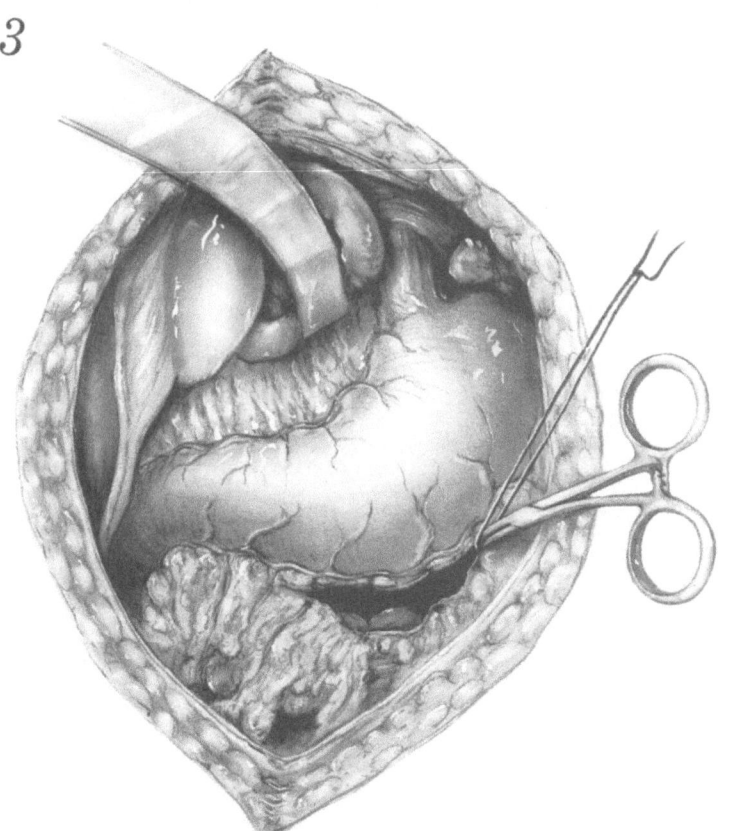

3 Mobilisation is commenced at the midpoint of the greater curve by dividing the greater omentum outwith the gastro-epiploeic arcades. In tying the epiploeic branches of this arcade care must be taken not to injure the parent vessels on which the vascularity of the stomach and anastomosis depends. Mobilisation should continue distally along the gastro-epiploeic arcade to the entry of the right gastro-epiploeic artery, which must be preserved. Mobilisation continues proximally along the greater curve, dividing the left gastro-epiploeic artery.

4

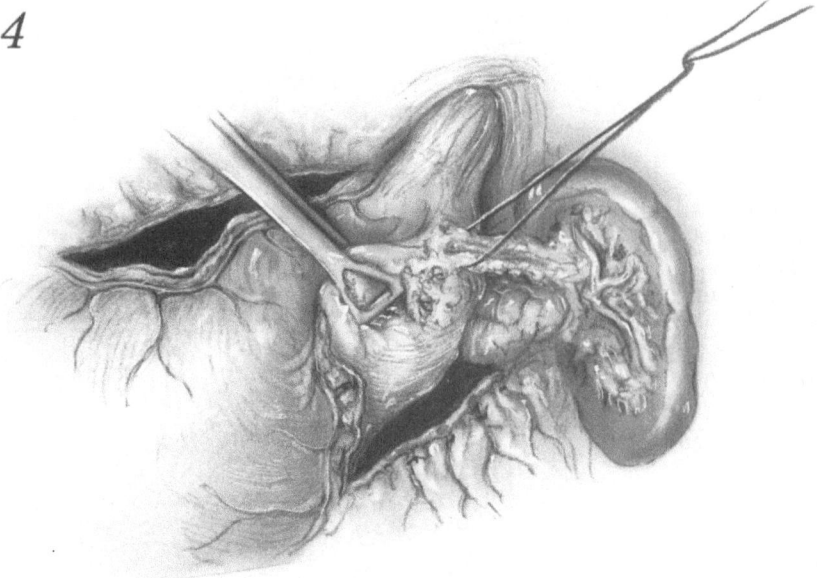

4 The short gastric arteries are identified and divided, taking care not to include the stomach wall. This mobilisation may be facilitated by rotating the operating table towards the patient's right and by drawing the fundus of the stomach inferiorly with a tissue forcep. Mobilisation of the greater curve should now be complete to the oesophageal hiatus. Mobilisation along the lesser curve divides the lesser omentum, taking care to identify any aberrant hepatic branches of the left gastric artery.

5

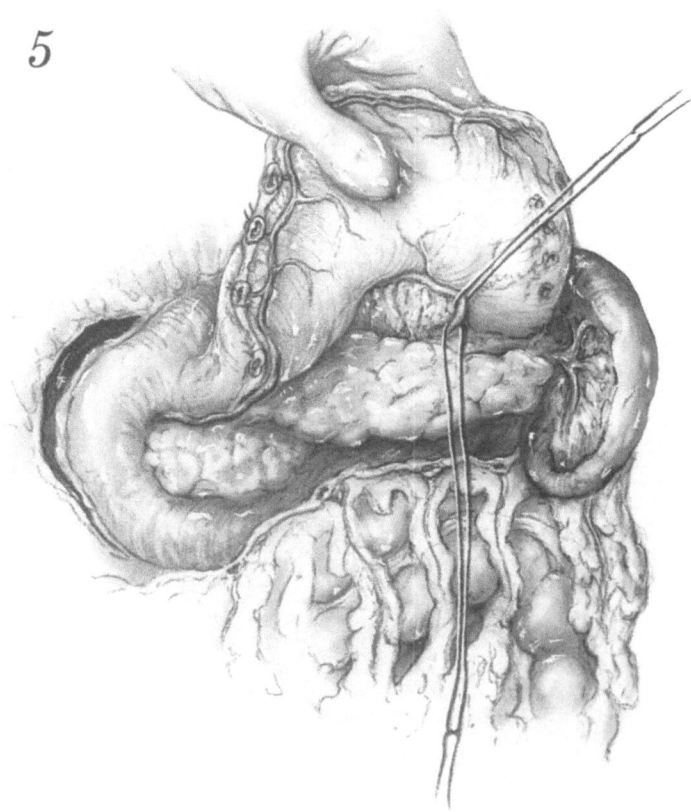

5 The mobilised stomach may now be lifted upwards, to identify the left gastric artery as it emerges from the upper border of the pancreas. It should be divided as close to the retroperitoneal wall as possible and double ligatures are recommended on the large, often atheromatous vessel.

6 The stomach is now completely mobile, anchored only by the duodenum, the right gastro-epiploeic and right gastric arteries and the oesophagus. A tape may be passed around the cardia and used to bring the oesophagus into the abdomen. Crushing clamps should then be applied across the oesophagus, which is then transected. The proximal stump of the oesophagus is transfixed with a non-absorbable suture and allowed to retract into the chest.

6

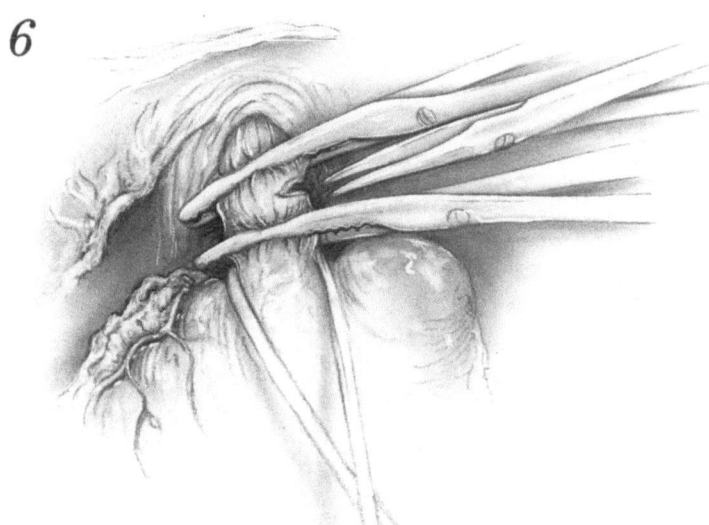

7

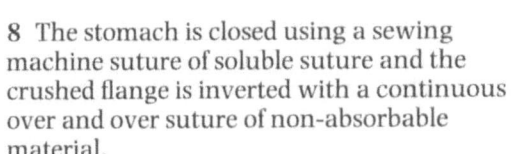

7 The gastric tube is then delivered onto the anterior abdominal wall. The oesophageal remnant and the gastro-oesophageal junction should be excised. A Peyr's crushing clamp is applied obliquely on the gastric side of the junction and the remnant is excised.

8

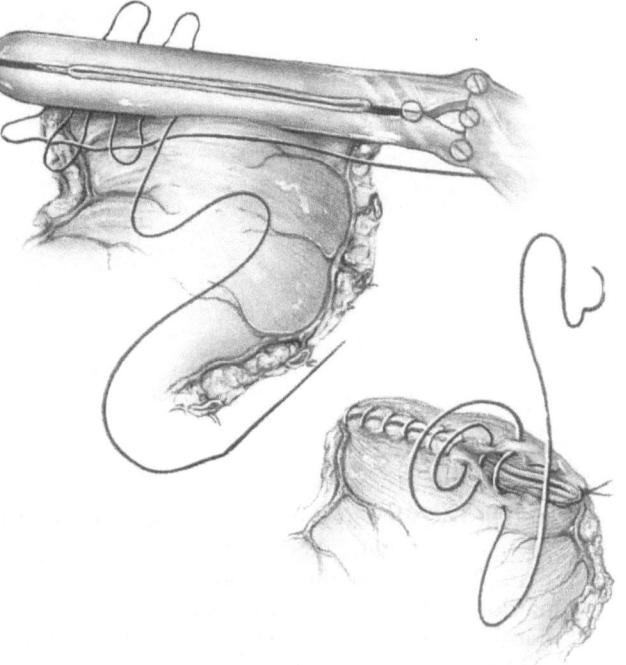

8 The stomach is closed using a sewing machine suture of soluble suture and the crushed flange is inverted with a continuous over and over suture of non-absorbable material.
If the pylorus is scarred a pyloroplasty should be performed.

9

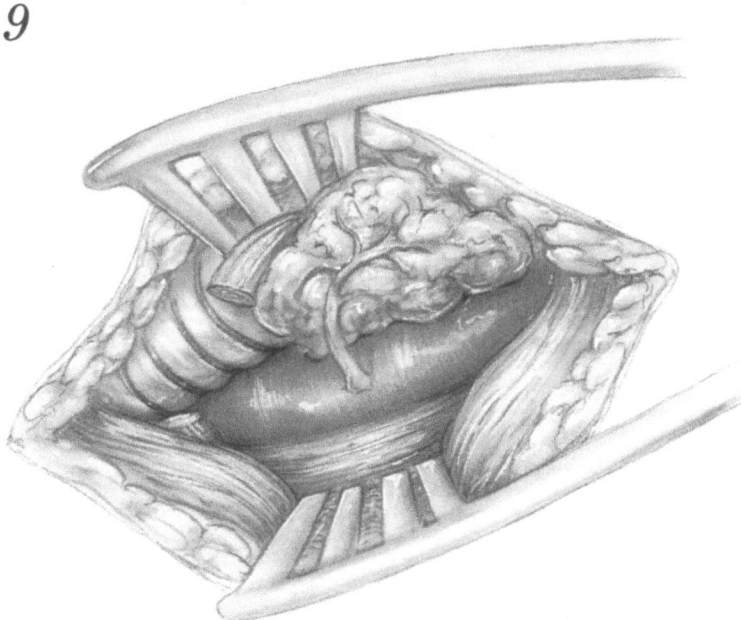

9 The neck incision is then performed on the side of the non-dominant arm, passing along the anterior border of the sternomastoid muscle. The dissection proceeds medial to the carotid sheath, dividing the middle thyroid vein and the omohyoid muscle.

10

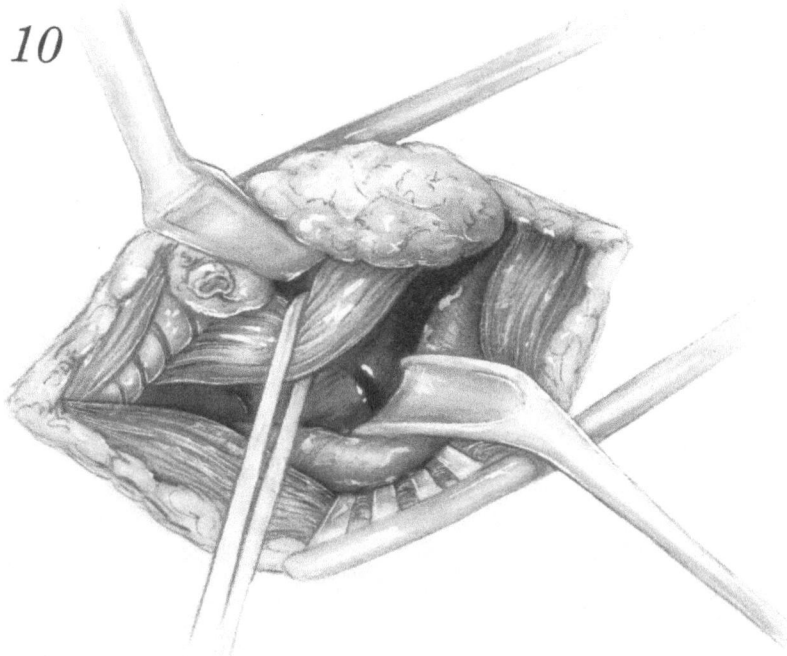

10 The oesophagus is identified, lying between the trachea and the prevertebral fascia. The left recurrent laryngeal nerve should be identified and a sling passed around the oesophagus, keeping close to its wall in an effort to avoid the contralateral recurrent laryngeal nerve. Blunt dissection may then be carried inferiorly into the thorax to mobilise the oesophagus, which is then clamped and divided at the lower margin of the dissection. The distal stump is transfixed with a non-absorbable suture and allowed to retract into the thorax.

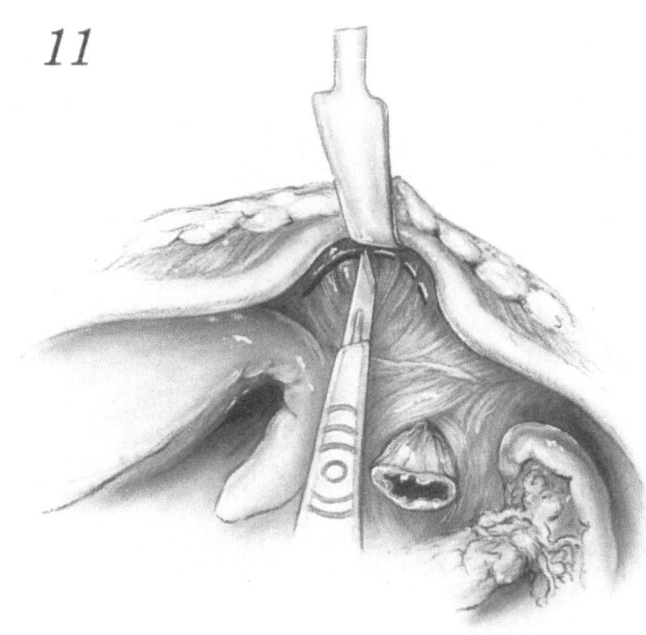

11 The surgeon returns to the abdominal dissection, the foramen of Morgagni is incised and blunt dissection creates a plane beneath the sternum, sweeping the left and right pleurae laterally. Either or both pleural spaces may be inadvertently opened at this stage and a chest drain may be required.

12

11

12 The substernal space developed easily accommodates the surgeon's forearm and he is then able to complete the dissection to the neck incision by blunt division of the fascial attachments to the sternum. Usually the thoracic inlet will not comfortably accommodate the gastric tube and so should be enlarged. The skin incision is extended onto the manubrium sterni, the sternomastoid muscle is reflected from its sternal and clavicular attachments, and the head of the clavicle, the sternoclavicular joint, and the upper and outer quadrant of the manubrium sterni are resected using large bone gougers.

13

13 The gastric tube is then carried through the substernal space to the neck dissection on the surgeon's hand, taking care that torsion does not occur. The stomach tube reaches with ease to the neck and there should be no tension on the vascular pedicle.

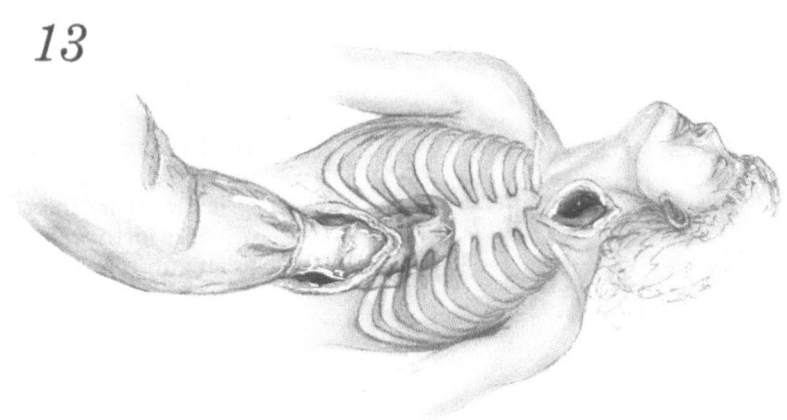

14

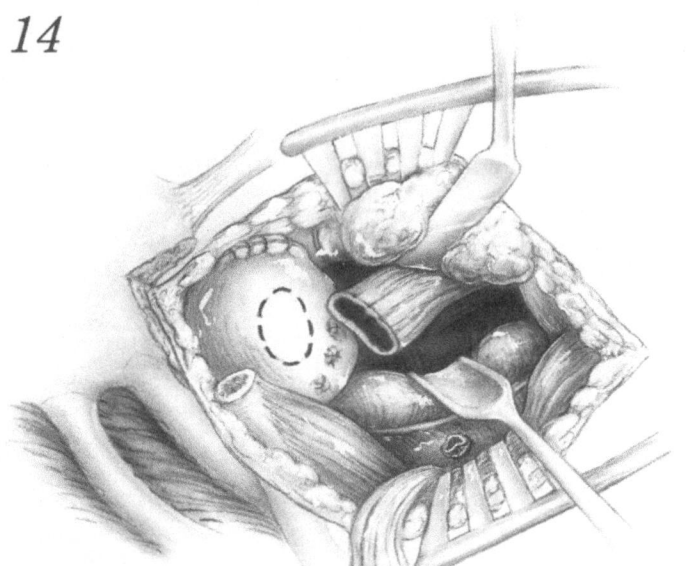

14 A suitable site for the anastomosis is identified on the fundus of the stomach, avoiding the gastric closure. A circular full thickness defect is created in the stomach, 2·5 cm in diameter. The submucosal plexus should bleed profusely and pinpoint haemostasis may be desirable. It is best not to attempt complete haemostasis and the anastomosis may be performed with some continued bleeding.

15

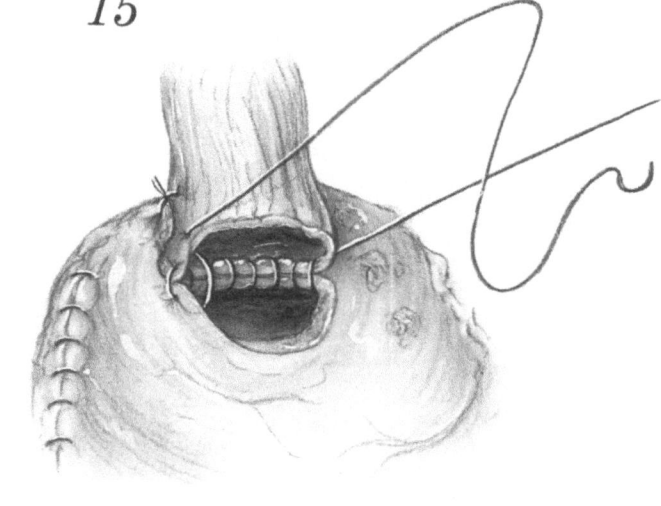

15 An end to side oesophago-gastric anastomosis is undertaken, using a single layer of continuous 3·0 monofilament non-absorbable suture, taking generous full thickness bites of oesophagus and stomach. If a nasogastric tube is required, it may be passed at this stage and negotiated into the stomach before the anastomosis is completed. The anastomosis may be facilitated by flexing the neck.

16

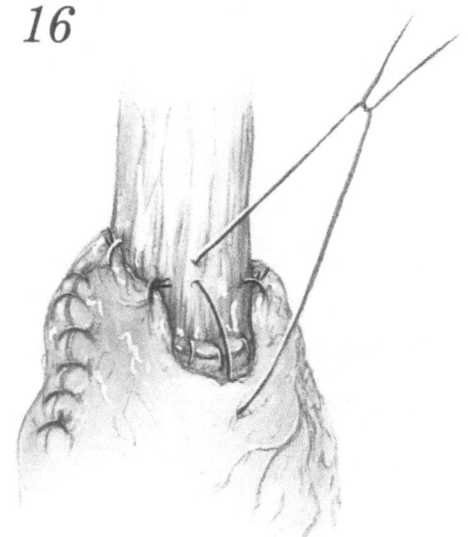

16 The stomach may be drawn up around the anastomosis, invaginating the oesophagus and fixing it to surrounding structures with interrupted non-absorbable sutures. This provides further support for the anastomosis and may function as an anti-reflux mechanism.

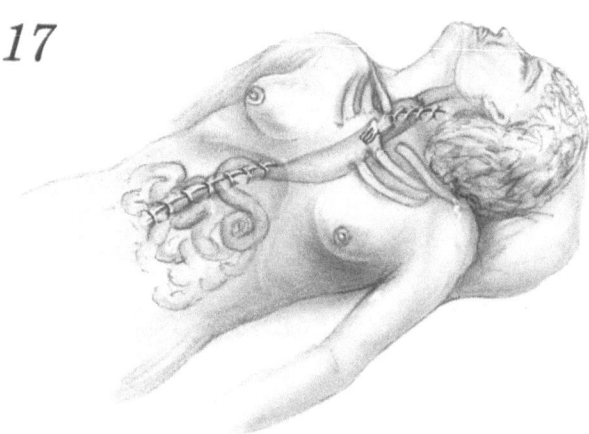

17

17 The abdominal closure commences with the peritoneum. The linea alba is closed using a continuous monofilament non-absorbable suture, taking care to bury the bulky knots. The closure is then completed by subcutaneous and skin closure. Before closing the cervical incision a corrugated drain is led from the region of the anastomosis through a separate stab incision. The wound is then closed in layers using continuous sutures of absorbable material.

Free reflux will occur after this operation and fatal aspiration pneumonia has occurred. The patient should be nursed 30° head up at all times, especially whilst being transported from the operating theatre and recovering from the anaesthetic. It is our routine to keep the endotracheal tube in place with the cuff inflated until the patient is back in the ward and fully conscious.

Prophylactic antibiotics should be discontinued after 24 hours.

Once gastric emptying is evident and bowel sounds return, usually on the second or third day, the patient may commence oral fluids.

The patient soon resumes normal diet. Small, more frequent meals are usually necessary for some months until the stomach resumes its reservoir function.